THE
PROBLEM
WITH
BREASTFEEDING

A personal reflection

James Akre

THE PROBLEM WITH BREASTFEEDING

A personal reflection

© Copyright 2006

Hale Publishing, L.P.
1712 N. Forest
Amarillo, Texas 79106-7017 (USA)
www.iBreastfeeding.com
(806)-376-9900
(800)-378-1317
International (+1-806)-376-9900

ISBN: 0-9772268-4-0
ISBN 13 digit: 978-0-9772268-4-9

Library of Congress Number: 2006926590

THE PROBLEM WITH BREASTFEEDING

A personal reflection

James Akre
Geneva, Switzerland

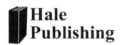
Hale Publishing

1712 N. Forest St.
Amarillo, Texas 79106 (USA)
www.iBreastfeeding.com

Dedication

I dedicate this book to seven remarkable women – Mary Ann Cahill, Edwina Froehlich, Mary Ann Kerwin, Viola Lennon, Betty Wagner Spandikow, Marian Tompson and Mary White – the co-founders, in 1956, of La Leche League International. Their combined compassion, vision and faith continue to radiate in 65 countries in the smiles of hundreds of thousands of three generations of children and mothers who have benefited from that fundamental form of self-help and mutual support that has been the League's trademark for the past half-century. Our world is a much happier, healthier place for their passing here. May the following reflection serve both to honor them and to advance their mission of helping mothers worldwide to breastfeed, while promoting a better understanding of breastfeeding's role in protecting children, mothers and society as a whole.

TABLE OF CONTENTS

ACKNOWLEDGEMENTS

Many individuals have contributed in big and small ways to the reflection that follows – some by helping me directly or indirectly in preparing it; others by inspiring me, whether through their unique contribution to the welfare of mothers and children or their own parenting style; and still others thanks to their greathearted mentoring. I recognize that reducing everyone's input to surface equivalence by listing names alphabetically, without comment, is inherently unfair. By the same token, I am confident that all concerned have a good idea how much their generosity, enthusiasm, intellectual rigor and friendship have marked my consciousness.

My sincere thanks go to Evi Adams, Elizabeth Aitken, Christina Akre, Daniel Akre, Pia Akre, Philip Akre, Nadida Altamimi, Alison Barrett, Mark Belsey, Sandra Lee Berner, Marie Biancuzzo, Monika Bloessner, Steve Chadwick, Graeme Clugston, Katherine Dettwyler, Claude Didierjean-Jouveau, Ros Escott, Ken Farmer, Elsa Freedman, Judith Galtry, Fiona Giles, Roberta Graham, Robin Gray, Karleen Gribble, Shirley Gross, Esther Goldstein, Rosemary Gordon, Anders Hakansson, Lars Hanson, Riripeti Haretuku, Anne Heritage, Sue Hobbs, Yngve Hofvander, Ewa Carlsson Höpperger, Elizabeth Hormann, Hilary Jacobson, Louise James, Yao Fei Juan, George Kent, Joanna Koch, Gisèle Laviolle, Virginia Leary, Janine Lewis, Rebecca Magalhaes, Laure Marchand-Lucas, Joanne Manchester, Chele Marmet, James McKenna, Patricia McVeagh, Dia Michels, Maureen Minchin, Catherine Minot, Philippe Minot, Pam Morrison, Gerald Moy, Barbara Mueller, Jack Newman, Arne Oshaug, Brian Palmer, Alberto Pradilla, Françoise Railhet, Alan Reilly, Mary Renfrew, Randa Saadeh, JoAnne Scott, Julie Smith, Linda Smith, Amy Spangler, Francine Strickwerda, Julie Stufkens, Azmara Tecle, David Tejada-de-Rivero, Janet Thomas, Anna Utter, Liz Weatherly, Diane Wiesinger, Barbara Wilson-Clay.

ABBREVIATIONS, ACRONYMS AND TERMS

AAP	American Academy of Pediatrics
ARA	Arachidonic acid
CBC	Canadian Broadcasting Corporation
CDC	Centers for Disease Control and Prevention (USA)
DHA	Docosahexaenoic acid
FAO	Food and Agriculture Organization of the United Nations
IBCLC	International Board Certified Lactation Consultant
IBFAN	International Baby Food Action Network
IBLCE	International Board of Lactation Consultant Examiners
ILCA	International Lactation Consultant Association
ILO	International Labour Organization
LCPUFA	Long-chain polyunsaturated fatty acids
LLLI	La Leche League International
NGO	Nongovernmental organization
Q&A	Question & Answer
RCP	Royal College of Physicians (Great Britain)
SIDS	Sudden Infant Death Syndrome.
UNICEF	United Nations Children's Fund
USDA	United States Department of Agriculture
WABA	World Alliance for Breastfeeding Action
WHO	World Health Organization
WIC	Supplemental Food Program for Women, Infants and Children (USA)

In the present context, the term:

- **"synthetic dream merchants"** refers to manufacturers and distributors of infant formula for routine non-emergency use;

- **"infant formula"** means an industrially prepared breast-milk substitute formulated in accordance with applicable FAO/WHO Codex Alimentarius standards to satisfy, by itself, the nutritional requirements of infants for the first months of life (precisely how long is a matter of continuing debate);

- **"hominid blueprint"** is the term anthropologist Katherine Dettwyler uses in the context of her research predicting age at weaning relative to various life-history variables, showing that extended breastfeeding is appropriate for our species. She has concluded from her research on correlates of weaning age in non-human primates – adult body size, length of gestation, timing of permanent tooth eruption, timing of sexual maturity, and growth rates during childhood – that modern humans should be breastfed for between two and a half and seven years;

- **"International Breastfeeding Support Collective"**, or Collective for short, is the virtual global organization I have imagined. Members are all voluntarily subscribing hominids of the species *Homo sapiens*;

- **"we"** usually refers to the members of the International Breastfeeding Support Collective.

All currency values are expressed in US dollars.

Reality must take precedence over public relations, for Mother Nature cannot be fooled.

Richard P. Feynman (1918-1988)
Nobel laureate in physics, teacher, storyteller, bongo player

I once knew a kangaroo[1] named Sue
That produced milk suitable for two.
Her left teats served lite
While those on the right
Provided hearty colostric brew.

James Akre (1944-   )
Observer of the human comedy, dabbler in doggerel and ardent fan of Mother Nature

---

[1] Kangaroos are the largest marsupial mammals. Females usually have one young annually and, as one more marvel of Nature, they take tailor-made nutrition for their offspring to dizzying heights. The joey remains in the pouch for nine months and continues to suckle until 12 to 17 months of age. Kangaroos can have three babies at a time: one maturing and just out of the pouch, another developing in the pouch, and one embryo in pause mode. There are four teats in the pouch and each provides different milk for different stages of development. Source: Kangaroo Facts http://www.giftlog.com/pictures/kangaroo_facts.htm.

GETTING STARTED

We all arrive in this world more or less the same way and in the same condition – naked, wet and hungry. After that, nearly all bets are off as culture kicks in and we begin the long differentiating journey to becoming who and what we are based on the rules of the group into which we're born.

This elementary observation of socialization's primacy is the basis for my abiding fascination with culture as a molding medium. It also accounts for my interest in the diversity of attitudes and practices surrounding a universal fundamental defining characteristic of our species – the nurturing and nutritional strategy called breastfeeding. But this wasn't always the case.

Growing up in the USA of more than a half-century ago in conditions of relative post-War abundance when breastfeeding rates were at an all-time low, the word breastfeeding wasn't part of even my passive vocabulary until my mid-teens. I recall being introduced to the notion of "eating to live" versus "living to eat". In time, particularly as a result of working in resource-poor settings in Africa, Asia and the Caribbean, I observed that, qualitatively speaking – with the exception of babies – for many people feeding had become an addendum to the main event: life and sustaining it. I saw this attitude reflected in popular adages like the Cameroonian pidgin English "Beli no dey get eye" – The stomach is blind, i.e. it cares only about being full; and the Haitian Créole "Sak vid pa kanp" – meaning, literally, an empty [jute or cloth] sack is unable to stand on its own, but with the metaphorical message that food, any food, is essential to sustain life and activity.

Traditionally, what we eat and the ceremony surrounding it depend on geography, climate and culture. While globalization is fast untying the first two nourishment knots in resource-rich settings, culture – modulated by economics – still reigns supreme in terms of food selection the world over. Not surprisingly then, our approach to the only true example of a universally common food and feeding system – breast milk and breastfeeding – continues to be conditioned by culture's stamp.

In contemplating the contemporary child-feeding horizon I conclude that many do not understand the implications of the biological norm for feeding the young of our species and the inherent dangers of deviating from it. I nevertheless remain optimistic that we can make a major improvement in child-feeding practices within a reasonably short time – even a single generation – if we are able to adjust appropriately the complex value system which determines whether society engages in more or less breastfeeding.

What follows is not intended as a convince-you text where breastfeeding as such is concerned. If, in the light of the compelling evidence that's readily available elsewhere, you don't already fully subscribe to breastfeeding's universal significance, it's unlikely that you will be won over by delving here.

On the other hand, if you already accept this fundamental truth, I hope that my reflection will contribute in two ways: by providing a different, or at least a less common, view of breastfeeding's cross-cultural commonalities and differences; and by suggesting what we might do, individually and collectively, to move things forward. Thus, rather than attempting to draw up an all-inclusive list of my intended audience, it makes more sense simply to say: everyone but non-subscribers.

Where breastfeeding is concerned, my most important teachers have consistently been my mother, sisters, wife, nieces, sisters-in-law, daughter-in-law, and colleagues and friends in the international breastfeeding community. I would like to thank them all for seeing so lovingly to my continuing education.

These are my most relevant credentials where the following pages are concerned. Like all readers, I am a mammal, and I have been since 1944. Then, like no doubt many readers, I am also a parent, in my case since 1974. More recently, like at least some readers, I am a grandparent and this since 2000. Lastly, once again like all readers, my individuality is based on the circumstances of my birth and the story of my life, which includes an international career in economic and social development and public health nutrition spanning four decades.

It is in this light that I would like to reflect in the following pages on a few of the lessons I have learned along the way and what I consider to be the most important implications for us as charter members of the International Breastfeeding Support Collective.

What's that, you say you're not yet a member of the Collective? Well, you're in luck!

The International Breastfeeding Support Collective is the ultimate member-friendly organization. The only qualifying credential is that you be a mammal of the species *Homo sapiens*. Beyond that there are no elected officers, no dues to pay, no meetings to attend and no newsletter to read. What's more, lifetime membership is yours for the asking. Just place your hand on your *breast* and repeat after me: "I am a mammal and I support breastfeeding unconditionally as an elemental act of allegiance to ourselves and to our children!"

There, that wasn't difficult now was it?

Oh, I almost forgot. You do in fact have one obligation after all. It's important for you to know that – borrowing from Seamus Heaney[1] – all members of the Collective automatically become ambassadors:

---

[1]Seamus Heaney, Nobel Prize Laureate in Literature (1995). From the Republic of Conscience http://thewitness.org/archive/march2002/poem.html.

The old man rose and gazed in my face
And said that was official recognition
that I was now a dual citizen.
He therefore desired me when I got home
to consider myself a representative
and to speak on their behalf in my own tongue.
Their embassies, he said, were everywhere.
but operated independently
and no ambassador would ever be relieved.

So, let's get started.

James Akre
Geneva, Switzerland
April 2006

Part one

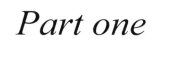

1. The problem with breastfeeding

I'll get right to the point. I don't have a problem with breastfeeding anymore than I presume anyone reading this paragraph does. But I do think that a significant portion of contemporary Western society does have a problem with breastfeeding, and that's mainly what I want to talk about. I would also like to suggest how we might look differently at the problem while altering our approach to doing something about it. We need to understand the breadth and depth of the current confusion about breastfeeding as a prelude to promoting the society-wide shift in awareness required to return it to its place of primacy in human development.

Breastfeeding remains a major unsolved riddle for many people, whether for the general population or health professionals and politicians. In a given sociocultural context, all are exposed to a similar set of values and attitudes – albeit with different outcomes – about this defining feature of our shared humanity. Despite the continuing avalanche of information in the popular and specialist media on the wonders of breast milk and breastfeeding, those of us who would alter perceptions about breastfeeding's universal lifelong significance continue to face a significant challenge.

I see the problem with breastfeeding as a source of particular perplexity, even distress, for many people under the Anglo-Saxon arc. I am using Anglo-Saxon in a limited colloquial sense to distinguish people and their common cultural roots, however diversely developed, found predominantly in Australia, Canada, Great Britain, Ireland, New Zealand and the USA, with degrees of overlay elsewhere, for example in parts of Africa, Asia and the Caribbean.

This is not to imply that other cultures don't exhibit similar dysfunctional attitudes toward breastfeeding. However, in addition to the Anglo-Saxon model being the one I know best, I see a key global dimension in this regard given its disproportionate influence on the rest of the world. By way of comparison, think about the impact of a single article of clothing – blue jeans – on popular culture the world over even as you reflect on the effect of fast-food – including infant formula – on how well populations fit into those jeans.

I've been considering the topic from a number of angles for four decades, and my single overriding conclusion is this: Where breastfeeding remains undervalued and under-practiced, the primary barrier to more and longer breastfeeding is society – wide ignorance both of human milk's unique, species-specific properties and of the inescapable implications for the health of all people throughout the life course. Moreover, this ignorance is as much a sign as it is a source of the disrespect for the biological norm for feeding the young of our species that contributes so effectively to ensuring a continuation of already low rates of breastfeeding prevalence and duration.

Every other barrier to breastfeeding – from individual attitudes and how they are formed, to non-supportive health services, to the multiple unhelpful ways society is often structured – can be traced directly to this cross-cutting core ignorance. And thus, to return breastfeeding to the realm of the ho-hum ordinary – which is how I define my goal for society – we also need a society-wide shift in awareness and attitude.

What I am saying can also be described this way. Contrary to the traditional view, I have concluded that it's not women who breastfeed after all; rather it's entire cultures and societies that do – or variously don't. In other words, cultures and societies *as a whole* are responsible for producing and sustaining the complex value system that results in more – or variously less – breastfeeding by the mothers and children in their midst. I base this observation on a single universal constant across time and geography: With only the rarest of exceptions, *all* mothers love their children and want what is best for them. And in terms of feeding behavior, "best" is invariably a culturally determined value.

We often talk about the role choice plays in our lives, which is understandable since we are fond of describing our behavior in terms of rational decision-making. But where child-feeding mode is concerned – to breastfeed or not – my sense is that it's roughly equivalent to the role that choice plays in deciding whether to hold a small child's hand as we cross a busy street together, which is to say not at all.

"I think I'll hold my six-year-old granddaughter's hand as we cross the street today, although frankly I'm getting a little tired of all this responsibility, so perhaps next time I'll just not bother."

Uh, no, not exactly.

We hold a small child's hand when crossing the street together because we know – as do the vast majority of people everywhere – that doing otherwise is irredeemably irresponsible, dangerous, culpable and downright stupid.

So, do we then "choose" not to breastfeed based on carefully worked out criteria? In the main, I think not. We respond the way we have *learned* to respond, which is why I insist that if we want to change a society's predominant artificial-feeding mode we need to change society in all its structural complexity – including an integrated production, transport, marketing, consumer, educational, social-welfare and health-care infrastructure, which itself is contingent on culturally determined expectations and behavior patterns – and not just focus on one or two contributing factors in isolation.

The breast-is-best mantra doesn't cut it anymore – if it ever did – in terms of preventing or reversing an artificial-feeding status quo. This should be obvious for several reasons, notably the fact that the very slogan "Breast is best!" has been so enthusiastically embraced by the synthetic dream merchants –

infant-formula manufacturers – who stand to profit most directly from perpetuating this status quo. As manufacturers continue to feint and feign with their damn praise, I suggest that we bear in mind Aesop's timeless caveat to his fellow Greeks more than 2,600 years ago (in *The fox without a tail*): Distrust interested advice!

If we are to reverse deeply rooted ignorance, a change in tactics is called for. We also need to pull apart and test our cherished assumptions about how we regard breastfeeding and the main stumbling blocks to making this fundamental survival strategy commonplace once again. Moreover, a critical eye is called for to see through the rhetorical fog, including the frequent and more or less sincere expression of the widespread belief that breastfeeding is somehow incompatible with being modern.

Said another way, I don't believe that we have either adequately asked, or successfully answered, the following key questions:

- Why do societies stray in the first place from the biological norm for feeding the young of our species?
- What continues to motivate many parents to defy the way children have been fed since pre-history?
- How is it that the synthetic dream merchants are so successful in securing their market share, at Mother Nature's expense, by promoting an alien food source for human babies?

It is less my intention to answer these questions directly than to use them as a backdrop and perspective for attempting to reconfigure the problem itself. And as you proceed, I would ask you to consider two additional points in this connection: the lessons we can learn by "stepping outside the box," that is borrowing from other areas of human experience to enrich our thinking and acting here; and what we can do better, differently or not at all to turn society around.

As noted earlier, my assumption is that readers are already convinced of the importance of breast milk and breastfeeding. Thus, rather than teaching you anything new in this connection my hope is to suggest alternative ways of looking at what you already know. As French essayist Marcel Proust remarked: "The real voyage of discovery consists not in seeking new landscapes, but in having new eyes."

2. Where do babies really come from?[1]

One day I ran a Google search using "where do babies come from" as key words. The result? I came up with no fewer than 4.4 million potential explanations of every possible description. In fact, my search was related to a report that I had read some years earlier about an interdisciplinary symposium organized in Paris under this intriguing title, which unexpectedly inspired the following reflection.

Notwithstanding first impressions, the Paris symposium was not on embryology or sexology. Rather, it was an opportunity for an international group of ethnologists, psychologists and psychoanalysts to discuss a question whose ultimate answer, finally, is not all that obvious.

Participants certainly examined the question from multiple perspectives, including science, the Devil, psychoanalysis, polytheism, our common primate heritage, and what medical science makes of all this.

And ample evidence was presented to shake a number of deeply held beliefs since the "real" answer to the question about where babies come from is forever linked to a specific culture and society. Whatever the precise response, it defines as much who we are as the rules governing our behavior.

So what does any of this have to do with breastfeeding? Well, that's at once easy and challenging to explain.

It's easy because, since prehistoric times, how babies *should* be fed has been a universal constant for our species.

---

[1]Adapted with permission from: Akre J. Les bébés, mais d'où viennent-t-ils vraiment? *Dossiers de l'allaitement*, Numéro hors série, Paris, La Leche League France, mars 1997.

It's challenging because of the way this basic biological imperative has been transformed – indeed *de*formed – in society. One thing is clear, however – it remains, first and foremost, a question of culture.

At birth nothing differentiates the sense of taste of a Nigerian or Peruvian baby from that of a Swiss, Canadian or Pacific-island baby. It's the "rules of life" that make the difference, the choices that are imposed by the group. And these choices not only affirm the group's overall identity; they define, more or less rigorously, how babies are cared for. More to the point in the present context, they also determine how babies are nurtured and nourished.

Generally speaking, choice in meeting human nutritional needs and the specific foods that are available and consumed depend on a variable mix of geography and culture. For this reason, apart from one exception it's no exaggeration to say that there is no such thing as a universal food. Naturally enough that exception is breast milk, which is the nutritional link par excellence for our entire human species – north, east, south and west – uniting as it does all 6.5 billion of us.

But if this is so, how is it that our common nutritional heritage is self-evident in some environments while it is regularly called into question – or simply ignored – in others?

And if feeding a baby initially anything other than breast milk remains a deviation from the biological norm for our species, how is it that this is so obvious for some yet so poorly understood by others?

Globally, the contrasts are striking indeed. For example, while more than 98% of babies throughout Scandinavia are breastfed as a matter of course, only one out of two babies in France and just four out of ten in Ireland ever see a drop of breast milk.

What's going on here? I'm tempted to suggest that the long-term "solution" to the problem lies in organizing six-month Scandinavian internships for the Irish and the French!

What then is a realistic way to approach this crucial cultural dimension? I believe that three observations are called for in this connection.

First, wherever breastfeeding takes a back seat to artificial feeding, it is highly improbable that the situation is going to be reversed without a strong push from the *bottom up*. Seven young mothers shared this visionary awareness 50 years ago and the founding of La Leche League International is eloquent abiding testimony to just how right they were.

Reinstating the primacy of breastfeeding requires stimulating sound judgment and finding new ways to educate mothers and fathers, children, extended families, health professionals, employers, trade unionists, governmental and political authorities, and many other individuals and groups throughout society. And this implies no less than a transformation of society in order to return to basic human values that will render breastfeeding normal, even ho-hum ordinary, once again.

Breastfeeding? But of course!

Singing the praises of breastfeeding while simultaneously resisting the siren song of the synthetic dream merchants (I'm referring to infant-formula manufacturers here) makes for a good start. But we also need to show that breastfeeding is not some sort of ideology to be defended; it is rather a universal act of allegiance to our children and to ourselves. We can do this by defining more clearly what is really at stake – for babies, children and adults, for mothers and families, and thus for entire societies – where both the short- and longer-term implications of appropriate or faulty child-feeding practices are concerned.

Second, it is imperative that we act in a manner that is consistent with who and what we are as a species, and that we strive to live in harmony with the basic laws – whether we attribute them to the Creator or to Mother Nature – that govern life itself.

Failing this, it is inevitable that we continue to suffer the consequences. Alarming reports abound in the scientific literature about the links between early consumption of cow's milk and risk of insulin-dependent diabetes; significantly higher blood pressure among adolescents fed formula as babies compared to their breastfed counterparts; and increased risk of obesity among children and adults who have been artificially fed.

Yet, these are just a few of the numerous negative implications, throughout the life course, of our collective impudence. We need to reconsider carefully the naturally dubious view that we are somehow able to deviate, with impunity, from our species' pre-established path, which has been evolving for many millions of years.

And third, we need to debunk a notion that, unfortunately, is far too common in the West as elsewhere – that being "modern" is somehow incompatible with breastfeeding. We need to remind ourselves that where this perceived inevitability is found, it is based first and foremost on society-wide ignorance of breastfeeding's true significance, and that this in turn translates into a lack of awareness also among young girls, women and mothers.

We should also realize that if this aspect of human behavior is to change, it needs to start with these very same young girls, women and mothers in the very same social environments in which they live and come of age rather than with any so-called higher political or public-health authority advising them. Commercial interests have long understood this reality; it is women consumers who decide and thus the objective is to convince women consumers.

These three observations are certainly not intended to increase the already heavy burden on the mothers of this world any more than they are meant to minimize the responsibility of other actors – including you and me – inside and outside the family.

The purpose is rather to recall the unique role, at once traditional and universal, that mothers play. In fact, it appears that this role is so obvious ... that it is often simply overlooked.

It is not only mothers who bring babies into the world, who nourish and teach them, but it is also mothers who are the first to transmit society's fundamental values.

Finally, then, isn't this the best way to reply to the question posed earlier: Where do babies *really* come from?

3. Whose right is it anyway?

Who has a right to breastfeed? Mothers only? Babies only? Children of any age? Mothers and children together? Well, I suppose it all depends on where you look and whom you ask.

Though most international human rights instruments don't mention breastfeeding explicitly, they do offer an inkling of enlightenment, starting with:

- the Universal Declaration of Human Rights (1948),[1] which states that "everyone has the right to a standard of living adequate for the health and well-being of himself and of his family, including food";
- the International Covenant on Economic, Social and Cultural Rights (1976),[2] which explicitly describes "the right to health" ("the enjoyment of the highest attainable standard of physical and mental health"), recognizes "the right of everyone to … adequate food," and notes that steps may be needed to ensure "the fundamental right to freedom from hunger and malnutrition" (as General Comment 12 on the right to adequate food (1999) observes: "The human right to adequate food is of crucial importance for the enjoyment of all rights."[3]);
- the Declaration of Alma-Ata (1978),[4] which calls health a human right and defines it as "complete physical, mental and social well-being, and not merely the absence of disease or infirmity".[5]

Article 24 of the Convention on the Rights of the Child (1989)[6] adds slightly to the picture and, in an encouraging development, explicitly mentions breastfeeding (albeit tepidly) for the first time in a global human rights instrument: "States Parties … shall take appropriate measures … to ensure that all segments of society, in particular parents and children ... are supported in the use of basic knowledge of child health and nutrition [and] the advantages of breastfeeding ..." Nevertheless, viewed from a purely chronological perspective – whether in terms of when the Universal Declaration of Human Rights was adopted or at what point breastfeeding begins – it's curious that not only did we have to wait 41 years for this first explicit mention; we also need to wade through the Convention's 600-word preamble and first 23 articles (out of 54) before we finally get to it.

The World Declaration on Nutrition (1992)[7] straightforwardly recognizes "that access to nutritionally adequate and safe food is a right of each individual"; and as a basis for the Declaration's accompanying Plan of Action for Nutrition and guidance for formulating national plans, governments pledged to "make all efforts to eliminate ... social and other impediments to optimal breastfeeding."

Okay, so most of these texts don't refer explicitly to breastfeeding, least of all to anyone's "right be to be breastfed." So what? How else are we going to approach the highest attainable standard of health and truly have access to nutritionally adequate food if we aren't breastfed? And how else are our children going to manage if they, too, aren't breastfed?

Some days I get the impression that there's a permanent stand-off between those who define breastfeeding as a child's "natural right" and those who adamantly speak only of a mother's "informed choice." You really have to love this latter expression, which borders on tautology – as if genuine choice were conceivable in the absence of a minimum of information from a disinterested source (cf. Aesop's caveat, chapter 1). I'm reminded of the impression that infant formula manufacturers give when they use these magic words: They do the informing while, on this basis, mothers are expected to do the choosing. In fact, if mothers were *genuinely* informed they would choose breastfeeding every time, as indeed would babies if they could because that's what they are naturally prepared to receive when they enter this world.

Meanwhile, even sympathetic human rights proponents are quick to caution breastfeeding advocates that a child's right to be breastfed is not explicitly recognized under international human rights law. After all, a *right* for one automatically implies a *duty* for the other doesn't it? (The fashionable human rights jargon "claim-holder" and "duty-bearer" might be useful elsewhere, but frankly I find these terms distinctly unhelpful in the present context. They seem to insinuate a mother/child adversarial relationship, as if between claimant and defendant in a judicial proceeding.)

Michael Latham describes as "strange, even aberrant" that the right to breastfeed is even discussed; he calls it a challenge to nature, to natural law and natural practice, and to our ecology and environment, and concludes that huge numbers of human infants not being breastfed and mothers being influenced not to breastfeed their babies is a distortion of nature (I agree fully on both counts). He also refers to mothers, who are not breastfeeding because of obstacles, as having suffered the loss of a right; he argues that, since "almost all mothers living under optimally baby-friendly conditions would make the choice to breastfeed," what is needed is action to remove obstacles to breastfeeding.[8] I consider this observation to be consistent with my own view that returning breastfeeding to the realm of the ho-hum ordinary requires a society-wide shift in understanding and motivation.

But Latham never really grasps the "mothers have a duty to breastfeed" nettle – and I certainly don't blame him for this – any more than the WABA Global Forum[9] did in 1996 when it included the following text in its recommendations:

> *Combined with the fact that breastfeeding is in the best interest of children and mothers, WABA interprets these general provisions of the Convention on the Rights of the Child as implying that children have a right to mother's milk as the only fully adequate food, and that mothers and children have a right to enjoy conditions that facilitate breastfeeding. States Parties have an*

obligation to respect, protect, and facilitate or fulfill the right to enjoy such conditions by the removal of obstacles to breastfeeding and to appropriate complementary feeding by the creation of supportive social and economic environments for parents and children. **This shall in no way be understood or perceived as the mother having a duty to breastfeed** *(emphasis added) since it is the circumstances which lead to the choice not to breastfeed that must be altered.*

George Kent also depicts the main task as removing the obstacles women face to feeding their infants in accordance with their well-informed choices rather than prescribing what they should do. In addition, he proposes that mother and child together be understood as having a type of group rights.[10]

Since both mothers and children breastfeed, by defining the breastfeeding twosome in terms of a right/duty relationship, we do indeed appear to be painting ourselves into a corner of classic dilemma proportions. Few politicians – and let's not forget that it's politicians who decide if and when the human rights bar is going to be raised – are prepared to tell mothers they have a *duty* to breastfeed their children.

Whose right is it then and how do we satisfy it for the one without infringing on the right of the other? Is it possible to tiptoe between the horns of a dilemma in a way that fully respects the individuality, integrity and rights of both parties?

Well, in my view we can begin by deliberately walking *away* from this pseudo dilemma. We don't need to butt our heads against a false conundrum; as some are presently defining it, this indeed becomes a zero-sum game, which automatically produces only one winner – and inevitably one loser – every single time.

We then need to decide what this particular win-win alliance is *really* all about – children and mothers whose health and welfare are simultaneously and mutually fostered, reinforced and protected, immediately and across the entire life course, thereby rewarding not only mothers and children but the entire society.

A joint right anyone?

When breastfeeding has been understood this way (and I have yet to fix a precise deadline for when this new regime will be fully in place!) we will be well on our way to appreciating that routine artificial feeding – as distinct from an exceptional emergency nutrition intervention – is the height of society-wide irresponsibility.

References
1. Adopted by the General Assembly of the United Nations on December 10, 1948.
2. Adopted by the General Assembly of the United Nations on December 16, 1966; entered into force January 3, 1976, in accordance with Article 27.
3. United Nations, Economic and Social Council, Committee on Economic, Social and Cultural Rights. The right to adequate food (Art. 11): 12/05/99. E/C.12/1999/5. (General Comments), paragraph 1. http://www.unhchr.ch/tbs/doc.nsf/0/3d02758c707031d58025677f003b73b9?OpenDocument.
4. World Health Organization/United Nations Children's Fund. International Conference on Primary Health Care, Alma-Ata, USSR, September 6-12, 1978.
5. These words are taken directly from the Preamble of the Constitution of the World Health Organization as adopted by the International Health Conference, New York, June 19-22, 1946; signed on July 22, 1946 by the representatives of 61 States (Official Records of the World Health Organization, no. 2, p. 100) and entered into force on April 7, 1948. This definition has not been amended since 1948.
6. Adopted by the General Assembly of the United Nations on November 20, 1989; entered into force September 2, 1990, in accordance with Article 49.
7. Food and Agriculture Organization of the United Nations/World Health Organization. International Conference on Nutrition, World Declaration and Plan of Action for Nutrition. Rome, December 1992.
8. Latham MC. Breastfeeding a human rights issues? *International Journal of Human Rights*, Special Issue on Food and Nutrition Rights, 1997: 5(4) http://www2.hawaii.edu/~kent/ijcr.htm.
9. World Alliance for Breastfeeding Action, WABA Global Forum on Children's Health and Children's Rights, Bangkok, December 2-6, 1996.
10. George Kent, PhD, University of Hawaii. Letter to the Editor. Response to "Breastfeeding and Human Rights" (J. Hum Lact. 2003;19:357-361), *Journal of Human Lactation*, 20(2), 2004.

4. Revolutions and counterrevolutions

If you were to ask me when I think the breastfeeding revolution is going to arrive, I'd respond that it's already here. The reason is simple really in its own complex sort of way, and I liken it to what I've experienced elsewhere. You see, I've already lived – or more accurately I'm still living – through a number of public health revolutions. Two obvious examples come to mind: the relatively rapid, radical and increasingly global shift, first in attitudes and then in behavior, toward using car seat belts and away from using tobacco products. And no matter how reasonable, even obvious, these changes appear in retrospect, I am also aware that both have had to drag in their path of change many of the kicking-and-screaming unconverted.

My earliest car memories as a kid were of Dad's 1948 cerulean blue Chrysler and our family doctor's canary yellow Pontiac – spiffy colors indeed in a predominantly various-shades-of-gray post-War America. Neither vehicle had seat belts of course; they hadn't been "invented" yet. So, if I was riding in the front seat next to Dad, he habitually extended his long right arm, palm spread wide against my pint-sized four-year-old chest, to prevent me from slamming into the dashboard, or worse, when braking.

I don't remember when I first used a seat belt as a passenger, but I clearly recall when I started using a seat belt regularly as a driver, to the point where I would have felt ill at ease riding unrestrained. I was 19 and during my last two years (1964-1966) as an undergraduate in Erie, Pennsylvania, I worked in a drugstore where part of my daily routine was delivering medicines to customers' homes using the boss's seat-belt equipped station wagon. Since then, I have hardly ever driven a vehicle without a seat belt, even if extending this elementary safety precaution to my own children two decades later turned into an unexpected challenge.

I bought my first car in Switzerland in 1974. Then-contemporary motor vehicle specifications meant that it came equipped with front seat belts only, even if the law didn't actually require their use until 1981. Meanwhile, an emotion-filled debate raged nationally for several years complete with political parties staking out positions, threats of a referendum to make obligatory (or not), and charges and countercharges from the pro and con camps swirling around safety versus individual liberty in the confines of one's own automobile.

The situation hadn't evolved much by the time I bought my second front-seat-belt-equipped car in 1980. I tried no fewer than six Swiss automotive spare-part dealers to find a set of rear belts for my children, who were six and four years old; no luck, though I was assured it would be possible to order directly from the Japanese manufacturer (I finally located a set in an Erie junkyard). By way of sociocultural footnote, my unsuccessful search for back-seat belts to secure my children's safety met with the identical incredulous response at all six spare-part dealers: "Why do you want to do that? The law doesn't require you to."

The arrival in the family of a third child in 1984 meant that a bigger car was needed, and what a relief it was to see that the law had been modified. All new cars now came equipped with front *and* rear seat belts (even if the law obliged only front-belt use). Then, gradually and grudgingly, law and practice began to change – like front belts in 1981, rear belts, too, had to be worn at all times from 1994; the political uproar ceased; and motorists, in the main, started to buckle up. Use rates for drivers climbed from 35% in 1980 to 82% in 2005, even if back-seat passengers trailed significantly (32% in 1995 to 53% in 2005).[1] I think it fair to say that the equivalent of a $15 fine (increased to $45 in 2005) for failure to buckle up was hardly a prime motivating factor. Rather, after a generation of political debate, resistance and ambiguity, most of the Swiss population – even people not wearing seat belts regularly – has finally internalized the why and the wherefore of this public health measure and begun to act accordingly.

John Cameron Swayze led the Camel News Caravan – Camel as in cigarettes – from 1948 to 1956, and Dad and I were both faithful followers. This was US network television's – and I presume the world's – first nightly news show sponsored by the R.J. Reynolds Tobacco Company, and Dad and I regularly watched it together.

Both my parents smoked, as did many adults of their generation including most of my aunts and uncles (of course I eventually lost my share of family members to smoking-related diseases). Mom smoked ladylike cork-tipped something-or-others, but Dad, being a man's man and an ex-Marine, smoked unfiltered Camels. The period 1940-1945 had been marked by a precipitous increase in adult smoking stimulated by WWII and large-scale tobacco consumption both by troops overseas and ever-increasing numbers of women at home. Lucky Strike Green may have gone to war – thanks to the hugely successful American Tobacco Company patriotic advertising campaign[2] – but Dad came marching home smoking Camels. Thus, well before I had taken my first puff I was already receiving a potent daily dose of positive emotional reinforcement – whether toward smoking in general or to Dad's brand in particular – as a defining feature of a treasured father-son ritual.

The era's seamless smoking-as-norm façade – or smokescreen if you prefer – started disintegrating soon enough. During my second decade of life I began the slow socialization shift away from smoking-as-good that partly paralleled some key dates in the history of anti-tobacco campaigning. These included:

- the first large-scale epidemiological study of the relationship between smoking and lung cancer showing that of 1,357 men so stricken 99.5% were smokers (1950[3]);

- the first widespread popular dissemination of evidence documenting the association between smoking and lung cancer (1952[4] and 1954[5]);
- the first biological link between smoking and cancer with a report that painting cigarette tar on the backs of mice created tumors (1953[6]);
- the first Royal College of Physicians (RCP) report calling for restriction on tobacco advertising, cigarette sales to children and smoking in public places (1962[7]);
- the first US Surgeon General's report on smoking and health that corroborated the RCP conclusions (1964[8]); and, a year after I left the USA,
- the first World Conference on Smoking and Health in New York with delegations from 34 countries (1967[9]).

The smoking-or-health history book also shows just how important tobacco company retrenchment, obfuscation and deceit were to prolonging for at least a generation the denial which shielded so many nicotine-addicted adults from accepting the awful truth: Smoking incapacitates and kills.

Looking back over the last half-century, the global results are remarkable indeed, whether in terms of action on the public health front or increased individual awareness within the general public. In the USA, for example, whereas 42% of adults (52% of men and 34% of women) smoked in 1965, by 2005 the figure had dropped to 20.9% overall.[10] In New York City alone, where the number of adult smokers dropped more than 100,000 in a year (21.6% to 19.3% from 2002 to 2003), surveys also found a 13% decline in cigarette consumption, suggesting that even smokers not quitting were nevertheless smoking less.[11]

Today, governments around the world are employing a variety of classic stratagems to curb tobacco use, for example price hikes, and sweeping bans on advertising and smoking in public places. At the same time, they are innovating with cigarette packets bearing graphic images of the damage done to internal organs by smoking (Canada), "de-normalizing" smoking as a social pastime (Norway), and justifying restrictions in bars and restaurants given the vulnerability of staff (Norway and Sweden). While smoking generates $65 million annually for Kenya's state coffers, it costs five times as much in disease, disability and death,[12] thus giving rise to a Government bill outlawing smoking in public places. In February 2006 the British Parliament voted for a full smoking ban in all pubs and clubs (a major poll in December 2005 found 71% in favor of making all workplaces smoke-free).[13] Even notoriously heavy tobacco-using countries like Ireland,[14] Italy[15] (followed by the Italian-speaking Swiss canton of Ticino[16]) and Spain[17] (the last with more than 50,000 smoking-related deaths annually[18]) have adopted remarkably stringent anti-smoking measures applicable to restaurants, bars, discos and nightclubs despite generally unfounded fears they would be widely flouted. Switzerland's largest retailer chose World No-Tobacco Day (May 31, 2006) to make all its 204 restaurants no-smoking.[19] Meanwhile, consistent with most of the world's commercial airlines, high-speed trains in France joined all trains in Belgium, Italy, Netherlands, Norway and Sweden by becoming smoke-free in December 2004[20] followed by Swiss trains a year later.[21] These examples are consistent with the growing international political will that culminated in May 2003 with adoption of the World Health Organization's Framework Convention on Tobacco Control,[22] which had achieved 107 ratifications by November 2005.[23]

The way I gauge things, the breastfeeding revolution – in fact counterrevolution is a more accurate descriptor – has not only already begun; it is also largely achievable within the space of a generation – *provided* we apply ourselves. I say this for a number of reasons, including:

- higher global breastfeeding rates, which have risen by at least 15% since 1990, and higher levels of exclusive breastfeeding for children under six months, which increased by as much as three- or fourfold in some low-income countries between 1990 and 2000;[24]

- 50 years of remarkably effective spadework by La Leche League, which now has 6,500 accredited leaders providing community-based support to more than 100,000 mothers every month in 69 countries;[25]
- improved standards of care thanks to the increasing number of International Board Certified Lactation Consultants (more than 24,000 candidates have sat the exam since 1985 and at present there are nearly 17,000 certified Consultants in 65 countries)[26] and to the International Lactation Consultant Association[27] (founded in 1985, ILCA now has 4,000 members in 50 countries on six continents);
- the nearly 20,000 hospitals in some 150 countries declared "baby-friendly" since 1991;[28]
- the worldwide activities of the International Baby Food Action Network (IBFAN)[29] and the World Alliance for Breastfeeding Action (WABA);[30]
- three decades of grass-roots and international political activism against unfettered merchandising of industrially prepared breast-milk substitutes;[31]
- an endless avalanche of scientific and epidemiological evidence repeatedly demonstrating both the incomparability of the biological norm for feeding the young of our species and the ravages wreaked on children and mothers alike by routine artificial feeding;
- continuing operation of nonprofit human-milk banks[32] and the opening of new ones in high-, medium- and low-income countries despite regular going-out-of-business forecasts in the age of HIV/AIDS;[33] and, to the dismay of some critics,[34] the advent of a sophisticated for-profit[35] operation in southern California[36] that is billed as "the first large-scale centralized facility for processing donor breast milk" in the USA;[37]

- adoption of legislation or other forms of protection guaranteeing a mother's right to breastfeed anywhere she otherwise has a right to be, including in New Zealand (the Human Rights Act[38] lists the areas of public life where the right to breastfeed is protected, although some critics don't feel it's enough); Scotland[39] (a campaign is under way to extend this protection elsewhere in the United Kingdom[40]); and, since Florida became the first to do so in March 1993,[41] in 32 of the 50 US states[42] with several others likely to take action soon (in the view of most people I know who are not from the USA, the only thing more outrageous than adopting such measures is the need to do so);
- reports of unconventional (and potentially risky) behavior suggesting growing awareness of breast milk's significance for human health, for example people surfing the Internet to buy, sell[43] or donate milk for babies[44] and cancer patients who are turning to breast milk in an attempt to boost their immune systems.[45]
- the fact that, thanks to WABA's global organizational skills and motivating abilities, millions of ordinary people now celebrate World Breastfeeding Week[46] every year in some 120 countries.

The cumulative result is growing popular, health-professional and political awareness of the significance of breastfeeding and breast milk, even if translating this awareness into increased prevalence and duration still has far to go in many settings. And while each of these points is a precondition to achieving the anticipated counterrevolution, my expectation is that it's the lingua franca of public- and private-sector budgets alike – the bottom line – that's finally going to trump most effectively non-emergency artificial feeding. Running the numbers successfully and understanding their significance accurately should serve as a tipping point for achieving the critical mass required to turn society's attitudes *and* behavior radically around based on a shifting sense of societal self-interest (see chapter 8). As with seat-belt and tobacco use, based on what we already know about the direct and indirect costs, to individuals and to society as a whole, of more or less breastfeeding, there should be no let up in promoting this health-enhancing behavior as an overall societal good. Breastfeeding is an idea whose time has returned. We quite literally can't afford to do otherwise.

But let me not appear to be waxing too lyrical too long. I am also keenly conscious of the challenge of change and its differential rate – slower or faster in one part of a culture or in one society compared with another. Public-health revolutions are anything but linear; despite real progress it's clear that in 2006 too many people still fail to buckle up and too many people still use tobacco in one form or another. But a key difference today is that virtually no one any longer dares to suggest that either approach is somehow beneficial or risk-free. Moreover, consensus about what is desirable, indeed normal, behavior in this regard could not be clearer.

Where breastfeeding is concerned, even if "everyone" supposedly now knows that breast is best, not nearly enough people know just how damaging routine artificial feeding is both for today's children and tomorrow's adults and the soaring price that society continues to pay for its collective ignorance. Postpartum child development, for better or for worse, is nutritionally programmed at the base level of still-maturing tissues and organs.[47] It is clear that achieving our genetic potential – including in terms of brain development, visual acuity, even longevity – is just not going to happen by ingesting a pediatric fast-food prepared from the milk of an alien species.[48]

Looking back over the last half-century, my sense is that while we still have a long way to go, we're already well into the breastfeeding counterrevolution. Compelling scientific and epidemiological evidence is available and being reinforced daily. We also have considerable experience with strategic thinking about what motivates populations to adopt or reject health-enhancing behavior.[49] But we need to move promptly – by restructuring society and culture, by bridging the gap between science and policy, and by using policy as a tool for improving public health[50] – to consolidate, expand and transform this knowledge into action that will take breastfeeding to the next plateau of significantly changed behavior.

Our awareness of breastfeeding's centrality in human development imposes additional responsibility to speak out. Now more than ever breastfeeding's future – and the speed and efficiency in molding it – depend on the members of the International Breastfeeding Support Collective. The Collective has its work cut out for it, no doubt about it. Moreover, it needs to be more aggressively focused on essentials, on which values draw the most members together, on developing a suitable language for expressing these values, and on communicating them effectively throughout society. Decrying the short-term harm of the excesses of multinational capitalism will never achieve the degree of attention of effectively communicating artificial feeding's disastrous impact on the health of children and mothers throughout the life course.

It's essential to remain big-picture strategists on the understanding that turning things around can happen only with a variety of tools, ideas and approaches employed synergistically. We need to take a closer look as much at what we are doing right or wrong as at what we are failing to do at all and what we might do differently that would make a difference. And because even grand strategies inevitably have unintended and unwanted consequences, we also need to be as quick-footed as we desire to be quick-witted. There is no magic bullet. As La Leche League's fifty-year worldwide experience amply demonstrates, at its most basic level success is measured one mother and one child at a time.

The highest remaining hurdles to more and longer breastfeeding are neither scientific nor epidemiological; they are primarily political, sociocultural, economic and organizational.

It's time to move more aggressively and sure-footedly on all four fronts. And as we do, let's not forget the singular advantage that we have over anyone who would still dare to promote a deviation from the hominid blueprint.[51] Embracing breastfeeding automatically places us on the right side of history.

References
1. Swiss Council for Accident Prevention. Statistics 2005, *Accidents in Switzerland* http://www.bfu.ch/english/statistics/2005/.
2. Lucky Strike Green Goes to War, 1942-1943 http://www.wclynx.com/burntofferings/adsluckystrikegreen.html.
3. Doll R, Hill AB. Smoking and carcinoma of the lung. Preliminary report. *British Medical Journal* 1950; 2:739-748.
4. Cancer by the carton. *Reader's Digest*, 1952.
5. The cigarette controversy, *Reader's Digest*, 1954.
6. Ernst L. Wynder, MD. *Morbidity and Mortality Weekly Report*, Atlanta. Centers for Disease Control and Prevention, November 5, 1999 http://www.cdc.gov/mmwr/preview/mmwrhtml/mm4843bx.htm.
7. Report of the Royal College of Physicians on Smoking and Health, 1962 (summary) http://www.ash.org.uk/html/policy/rcp40threport.html#_Toc3198703.
8. History of the 1964 Surgeon General's Report on Smoking and Health http://www.cdc.gov/tobacco/30yrsgen.htm.
9. Action on Smoking and Health http://ash.org/victories.html.
10. Lower adult smoking rates with more adults quitting. Levels still below nation's goal for 2010. Press release, November 10, 2005, Centers for Disease Control and Prevention, Atlanta, http://www.cdc.gov/od/oc/media/pressrel/r051110.htm.
11. Pérez-Peña R. A city of quitters? In strict New York, 11% fewer smokers. *The New York Times*, May 12, 2004 http://www.nytimes.com/2004/05/12/nyregion/12SMOK.html?ex=1399694400&en=e5f55c92a045a1f9&ei=5007&partner=USERLAND.
12. Smoking curbs: the global picture. BBC News, October 26, 2005 http://news.bbc.co.uk/1/hi/world/3758707.stm#europe.
13. UK smoking ban – Macmillan delighted at MPs' life saving action. *Medical News Today*, February 16, 2006.
14. Public Health (Tobacco) Act, 2002 (Section 47) Regulations 2003 http://www.irishstatutebook.ie/ZZSI481Y2003.html.
15. Italy bans smoking in public places, European Public Health Alliance, January 11, 2005, http://www.epha.org/a/1630.
16. Swissinfo. Smoking ban blazes a trail in Ticino, March 12, 2006.

17. Lawmakers approve definitive smoking ban. *International Herald Tribune*, December 16, 2005.
18. McLean R. For Spaniards, ashtray beckons. *International Herald Tribune*, December 29, 2005, page 1.
19. Migros Magazine, No. 13, March 28, 2006.
20. Rail Europe, press release http://www.raileurope.com/us/about_us/press_releases/nonsmoking_tgv.htm.
21. Swiss trains become smoke-free zones, the latest in a Europe-wide trend. News Blaze http://newsblaze.com/story/2005121510213100002.mwir/newsblaze/SMOKING1/Quit-Smoking.html.
22. The WHO Framework Convention on Tobacco Control. Geneva, World Health Organization, http://www.who.int/tobacco/framework/en/index.html.
23. The past and future of the WHO Framework Convention on Tobacco Control. Geneva, World Health Organization, http://www.who.int/tobacco/communications/events/seminar_10Nov05/en/index.html November 10, 2005.
24. UNICEF, Innocenti Research Centre, press release, November 22, 2005.
25. See La Leche League International http://www.lalecheleague.org/ for numerous links to national and regional affiliates.
26. The International Board of Lactation Consultant Examiners, Falls Church, Virginia, USA http://www.iblce.org/, administered its twenty-first annual credentialing examination in lactation consulting in July 2005. The test was administered in seven languages (for a total of 13 since 1985) to 2683 candidates in 135 locations across 32 countries and territories on 5 continents.
27. International Lactation Consultant Association http://www.ilca.org/.
28. World Health Organization/United Nations Children's Fund. Celebrating Innocenti 1990-2005. Achievements, challenges and future imperatives, 2005.
29. With regional coordinating offices in Africa, Asia/Pacific, Europe, Latin America/Caribbean and North America, the International Baby Food Action Network http://www.ibfan.org/ (IBFAN) consists of more than 150 groups worldwide http://www.ibfan.org/.
30. The World Alliance for Breastfeeding Action (WABA) http://www.waba.org.my/, founded in 1991, is a global network of organizations and individuals who believe that breastfeeding is the right of all children and mothers and who dedicate themselves to protecting, promoting and supporting this right.
31. See IBFAN http://www.ibfan.org/.

32. For example, in the Americas there are 168 human-milk banks in Brazil, 8 in Venezuela, 1 in Uruguay (http://www.paho.org/English/DD/PIN/ptoday19_sep05.htm) 1 in Canada (there were as many as 23 at one time but a tainted-blood scandal and concerns about spreading infections resulted in the closure of all but the Vancouver bank) and 9 in the USA (Human Milk Banking Association of North America http://www.hmbana.org/). Banks are also found in Bulgaria, Czech Republic, Denmark, Finland, France, Germany, Greece, India, Japan, Norway, South Africa, Sweden, Switzerland and the United Kingdom (http://www.lalecheleague.org/llleaderweb/LV/LVAprMay00p22.html). Australia's first human-milk bank is being established in 2006 at Perth's King Edward Memorial Hospital and another is expected to open soon in Queensland.

33. Pelgrim R. Milk of human kindness overflows. *Mail & Guardian Online* (South Africa), January 31, 2006.

34. Ensor D. Land of milk and money. *Paramus Post* (Paramus, New Jersey), March 27, 2006.

35. The largest nonprofit milk banks in the USA are reported to have distributed 745,329 ounces (more than 22 million ml) of milk in 2005 – double the amount in 2000 – at a cost of $2.6 million. In August 2005 Prolacta Bioscience http://www.prolacta.com/ started marketing a breast-milk concentrate for $48 an ounce (29.57 ml). Breast-milk trade sparks safety debate. *The Denver Post*, March 25, 2006.

36. SanDiego.com, *Land of milk and money*, February 12, 2006.

37. IOL, News for South Africa and the World. *Got milk? Want to sell it?* November 8, 2005.

38. Human Rights Commission. Human Rights in New Zealand Today. 4. The right to breastfeed. http://www.hrc.co.nz/report/chapters/chapter19/issues04.html.

39. Queen's Printer for Scotland. Breastfeeding etc. (Scotland) Act 2005 http://www.opsi.gov.uk/legislation/scotland/acts2005/20050001.htm.

40. UNICEF UK Baby Friendly Initiative. Westminster debates public breastfeeding bill, November 29, 2005 http://www.babyfriendly.org.uk/mailing/updates/news_update_20051129.htm.

41. Breastfeeding: gearing up for letting down. *Mothering*, Winter, 1993.

42. Adcox S. Breast-feeding rights bill clears [South Carolina] Senate, ready for [Governor] Sanford to sign. The State.com, April 5, 2006.

43. In the USA, where only two states – California and Texas – require breast-milk distributors to be licensed as milk banks, some mothers are selling their own milk on the Internet for $1 to $2.50 an ounce (29.57 ml). Breast-milk trade sparks safety debate, op. cit.

44. WSBTV.com, Atlanta. Jim Strickland investigates Internet breast milk. March 9, 2006; CNN.com. Not your mother's breast milk, January 26, 2006; Muñoz S. Mothers who share breast milk: Internet fuels movement aimed at supplying moms unable to nurse on their own. *Wall Street Journal*, January 4, 2005. Since January 2006 "one popular Web site has listed more than 100 human-milk advertisements". Got breast milk? Buyers are willing to pay. But booming trade raises safety, ethical questions. StarNewsOnline, March 26, 2006.

45. BBC News. The man who swears by breast milk, January 23, 2005; The WBALChannel.com, Can breast milk help treat cancer? Swedish researchers investigating milk's effect, February 28, 2006; The BostonChannel.com, Can breast milk help fight cancer? Doctor says larger effectiveness study needed, March 16, 2006.

46. First organized by the World Alliance for Breastfeeding Action (WABA) in a handful of countries in 1992 http://www.waba.org.my/.

47. Koletzko B, Akerblom H, Dodds PF, Ashwell M. *Early nutrition and its later consequences: new opportunities. Perinatal programming of adult health.* New York, Springer, 2005 http://www.danoneinstitute.org/publications/book/pdf/Book_Koletzko_ISBN_1402035349.pdf.

48. In multivariable analyses of the early life determinants of childhood intelligence in a population-based birth cohort of individuals born in Brisbane, Australia, the strongest and most robust predictors of intelligence were family income, parental education and breastfeeding, with these three variables explaining 7.5% of the variation in intelligence at age 14. Lawlor DA et al. Early life predictors of childhood intelligence: findings from the Mater-University study of pregnancy and its outcomes. *Paediatric and Perinatal Epidemiology*, 2006, 20(2):148-162.

49. See the Ottawa Charter for Health Promotion, World Health Organization, 1986 http://www.euro.who.int/AboutWHO/Policy/20010827_2.

50. Brush CA et al. Meeting the challenge: Using policy to improve children's health. *American Journal of Public Health*, 2004, 95(11):1904-1909.

51. Dettwyler KA. A time to wean. The hominid blueprint for the natural age of weaning in modern human populations. In: Stuart-Macadam P, Dettwyler KA (eds.), *Breastfeeding: biocultural perspectives*. New York, Aldine de Gruyter, 1995.

Part two

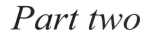

5. The Lactation Chronicles

American science fiction writer Ray Bradbury (b. 1920) is perhaps best known for his loosely knit 1950 short-story collection, The Martian Chronicles. The norm in science-fiction writing is for Earth to be invaded, as for example in H.G. Wells' classic War of the Worlds. Bradbury's book is thus something of an anomaly recounting as it does the invasion of Mars by refugee humans from a troubled Earth and the ensuing conflict between the colonized Martians and the colonizing Earthlings. As in Wells' classic, the Martians are killed off by Earth's bacteria; in the process, a wise and ancient civilization is destroyed. The work's title, premise and structure lend themselves as a fertile metaphorical leitmotif for the random opportunistic assemblage of the merely interesting, occasionally encouraging, just curious, frankly weird and – in terms of who we are as a species – the sometimes exceedingly alien accounts that follow here in log-like fashion. My purpose is to illustrate with real-world examples a number of the points made elsewhere in this volume about attitudes toward breasts, breastfeeding and breast milk. And just as comics are fond of assuring their audiences, I swear I'm not making up any of this stuff. Or to borrow from the timeless words of political cartoonist Walt Kelly (1913-1973), who believed that we are all responsible for our myriad pollutions, public, private and political: We have met the enemy and they are us.[1]

February 27, 2004. Darwin, Australia. Top down or bottom up?

A row erupted today over a police ban on traditional Aboriginal women doing as they have always done for the past 70,000 years – dance topless in public.[2] Aborigines are furious that a group of traditional women were moved on by police, including an Aboriginal officer, from a public park in Alice Springs last week because they were dancing without their tops. The women pointed out that dancing topless is part of Aboriginal culture, and anyway millions of people around the world had already seen them dancing like that on television, such as at the opening ceremony for the Sydney Olympics in 2000. Undeterred, a troupe of topless Aboriginal dancers welcomed Britain's Prince Charles to Alice Springs in March 2005.[3]

May 11, 2004. New York City. Mamma mia!
The New York *Daily News*[4] reported that a video installation about breastfeeding was removed from the "Sweet and Sour" art exhibition at the Fifth Avenue outlet of Italian luxury clothier Salvatore Ferragamo after a complaint from someone within the organization. Ferragamo commissioned works from selected artists inspired by objects in the store. The show promised to be "a fashionable exhibition of provocative paradoxes." Indeed. Artist Amy Jenkins' 20-minute video showed her, using a very discreet cradle hold, breastfeeding her 18-month-old daughter, who is sporting only a pair of the clothier's red Mary-Janes.[5]

May 21 & 24, 2004. London, England. No tit for some EU tat
The headline in London read "No nipples, please, we're British as breastfeeding film is censored"[6] while that in Sydney announced "Nipple causes ripple in the land that invented Page 3 girls."[7] Both reports concerned less than five seconds of a 45-second film promoting voting in the 2004 European Parliament elections; to show people making choices, like voters at the ballot box, it showed a suckling baby trying to decide which breast to feed from. The original version was considered suitable for nearly 400 million Europeans, and thus shown on television and in thousands of movie theatres in 23 countries. In Britain, however, where bare breasts are a daily staple in tabloid newspapers, the breastfeeding sequence survived but shots of the offending nipple were edited out by having the baby's hand obscure it. A spokesman at the Cinema Advertising Association defended the

censorship this way: "The infant was contemplating the breasts in rather an adult way." But at least the film was shown, unlike in Ireland where the head of the European Parliament's Irish Office, Jim O'Brien, was quoted as saying: "I decided that due to sensitivities here, this is not the right image to promote anything in Ireland, unless it is of a medical or scientific nature."

June 13, 2004. Sydney, Australia. Church group not playing around

Mothers at the weekly playgroup run by Saint Peter's (Cooks River) Anglican Church were told that they "might offend passing tradesmen or ethnic groups if they continue to breastfeed in the main hall, where their children play." A group of the women left the playgroup in disgust at the edict, which they labelled discriminatory and regressive.[8]

August 1, 2004. Auckland, New Zealand. Babe in arms: adults only

Women's Health Action[9] in New Zealand prepared a 15-second television ad to run during World Breastfeeding Week August 1-7, 2004. It depicted a girl, probably 8 or 9 years old, pretending to breastfeed her doll. A boy of similar age came into shot and said "Yuk, that's disgusting!" followed by an adult male voice-over saying "Isn't it time we all grew up?" The Television Commercial Approvals Bureau decided that it was "unsuitable for viewing by children under eleven" (it was permitted to run in the evening). The Bureau's general manager described the advocacy message as being aimed at modifying adult behaviour or views; the Bureau's concern was that it was using a negative situation to make a positive point but that many children would not understand the positive tag in the end message.[10] On the other hand, perhaps this would have provided a learning/teaching moment by stimulating at least some children to discuss the ad with their parents.

January 27, 2005. Geneva, Switzerland. To the breast of health (1)

Holly Abrams, Ph.D.
Scientific Director
HC Search Corporation
480 Second Street East
Ketchum, ID 83340-4991
USA

Dear Dr. Abrams,
Please accept my warm congratulations for your well-designed site on breast health and breast cancer http://www.healthsearches. org/. No doubt this will quickly become a welcome resource for members of the health professions and the general public alike. When consulting your site's Q&A section, however, I was struck by the absence of even an oblique reference to the importance of breastfeeding for preventing breast and other cancers … I trust that steps will be taken soon to integrate this important information in your website.

James Akre
Geneva, Switzerland

January 27, 2005. Ketchum, Idaho, USA. To the breast of health (2)

Dear Mr. Akre:
Thank you for your response and interest in our website … We at Healthsearches recognize breastfeeding as an important factor in reducing the risk of breast cancer in women. If a person searches under the key words "breastfeed," "breastfed" or "nursing," they will find that our website has several Q&A discussing the preventative benefit of breastfeeding. These Q&A are under the two subcategories called: Breastfeeding and

Risk and Controllable Risk Factors … In addition, we currently are expanding our Q&A section, including adding more topics about lactation and breastfeeding. Moreover, even in the first issue of our new magazine-style newsletter, *The Newsletter on Breast Health & Breast Cancer*, the cover article contrasting the incidence of breast cancer in Japan and the US mentions that breastfeeding can lower the risk of breast cancer …

Holly Abrams, Ph.D.
Scientific Director
Healthsearches

January 30, 2005. Geneva, Switzerland. To the breast of health (3)

Dear Dr. Abrams,

Thank you for your rapid and informative response to my message concerning breastfeeding's role in reducing the risk of breast cancer … Perhaps it's a question of perspective, whether the reference … belongs more appropriately under "prevention" or "risk" in the context of your elaborate Q&A. Personally, I see it as being relevant to both ... There is something especially attractive, reassuring, even empowering about the accessible answers provided to the very first question "Is there anything I can do to prevent breast cancer?" Moreover, while it is always possible to search for specific information relating to breastfeeding's protecting role, some readers will be left out simply because they don't know what they don't know in this connection. Surely, in the overall context of what an individual mother can do to protect her own health, even as she enhances that of her baby, breastfeeding deserves at least a *brief* mention in the first list, perhaps with a cross-reference to the section on risk reduction "for more information."

James Akre

February 13, 2005. Ketchum, Idaho, USA. To the breast of health (4)

Dear Mr. Akre:
We appreciate your continued interest in our website … Q&A on the benefit of breastfeeding in reducing the risk of breast cancer now can be found under both categories of prevention and risk. In the near future, we will be adding other Q&As on other benefits of nursing for the mother and benefits the breastfed child receives. In these Q&A on general benefits of breastfeeding, we will mention that organizations such as La Leche League International provide helpful information and support breastfeeding.

Holly Abrams, Ph.D.

February 13, 2005. Geneva, Switzerland. To the breast of health (5)

Dear Dr. Abrams,
I am grateful for your having responded as you did … These are surely important steps in the right direction … Adding a link to La Leche League International, the world's premier mother-to-mother support group now active in more than 60 countries, is also very positive. It is nevertheless disheartening to read the closing invitational proviso – in the answer to "If I breastfeed my baby, will that help prevent me from getting breast cancer?" – that:

> *In addition to helping reduce the risk of breast cancer, breastfeeding has other benefits. Nevertheless, if nursing your baby is not what is best for you and you infant, **the stress of nursing might be more damaging in the long run**. When considering breastfeeding, **weigh potential disadvantages and various benefits** of nursing your infant* [emphasis added].

Might be more damaging in the long run to whom and why? Surely, your site wants to be sensitive to the ambient US culture to which it is presumably mainly directed, although its potential impact is doubtless as wide as the Web itself. But in the light of available evidence, it just seems so unnecessarily soft, even wishy-washy, to close the section this way. And speaking of cultural relevance, although there are many good sources of up-to-date information and references, the most recent statement from the American Academy of Pediatrics on Breastfeeding and the Use of Human Milk[11] is perhaps a particularly useful link ... It just seems to me that the existing scientific and epidemiological evidence permits ... your site to be more enthusiastic about breastfeeding than it presently is.

James Akre

February 17, 2005. Ketchum, Idaho, USA. To the breast of health (6)

Dear Mr. Akre:
You are correct that the scientific and medical evidence is overwhelmingly in favor of healthy women breastfeeding their infants. We have revised the wording of the following two Q&A in the Prevention and Risk categories, respectively:
- Breastfeeding and Prevention of Breast Cancer
- Breastfeeding and Reduction of Risk of Breast Cancer

These two revised Q&A now:
- Reflect a more positive, empowering attitude towards breastfeeding
- Cite references including the policy statement of the American Academy of Pediatrics on "Breastfeeding and the Use of Human Milk"

- Recommend that women considering breastfeeding consult www.lalecheleague.org, the website of La Leche League International, which provides helpful information and support

Furthermore, we have added the following two new Q&A to the Prevention category:
- Breastfeeding and Relative benefits for the Child
- Breastfeeding and Relative benefits for the Mother

These two new Q&A on the benefits of breastfeeding:
- Reflect a positive, empowering attitude towards breastfeeding
- Cite references including the policy statement of the American Academy of Pediatrics
- Recommend that women considering breastfeeding consult www.lalecheleague.org

The Links section of our website is intended to feature advocacy and support groups as resources for people concerned about breast health and breast cancer. Would mutual links between the website of La Leche League International and the Healthsearches website be feasible? Please feel free to contact me.

Holly Abrams, Ph.D.

February 21, 2005. Ketchum, Idaho, USA. To the breast of health (7)

Dear Mr. Akre:
May I thank you again for your continued interest in the Healthsearches website on breast health and breast cancer ... Several of our Q&A on breastfeeding have been revised to reflect information in the updated guideline and now cite the 2005 AAP policy statement. These Q&A include the following topics:

- Breastfeeding and Prevention (of Breast Cancer)
- Breastfeeding and Reduction of Risk (of Breast Cancer)
- Breastfeeding: Relative benefits for the Child
- Breastfeeding: Relative benefits for the Mother

I have enjoyed your thoughtful correspondence and hope you will keep in touch as our website and newsletter evolve in the future.

Best wishes,
Holly Abrams, Ph.D.

April 13, 2005. Wellington, New Zealand. Ain't that a shame

There were numerous media reports in 2004 about La Leche League mother, Liz Weatherly, who was prevented from breastfeeding her two-and-a-half-year-old son in the entrance hall of a private preschool in suburban Auckland. Not only did she change schools for her son; in March 2005 she also presented a petition to Parliament with nearly nine thousand signatures calling for "action to address the lack of protection of the rights of breastfeeding women and children."[12] The Parliament's health committee agreed and formally recommended changes to existing legislation to explicitly protect breastfeeding. Also, the New Zealand Human Rights Commission organized a one-day forum in May 2005 to discuss principles for protecting breastfeeding rights. This is good news, of course, though I find distasteful the Commission's reference to overcoming the "social stigma" surrounding breastfeeding.[13] Do you really think that mothers are happy with breastfeeding linked to a word that means a "symbol of disgrace or infamy"? What a perverse way to describe this elemental act of allegiance to our species! A close second in the Perversity Sweepstakes: Government's choice of World Breastfeeding Week 2005 to announce that it *did not accept* the health committee's recommendations.

April 24, 2005. Raleigh, North Carolina, USA. Stick 'em up! Your formula or your life!

The first report[14] I saw concerned about $10,000 worth of cigarettes and hundreds of cans of infant formula stolen during an early morning break-in at a downtown Raleigh market. Powdered baby formula, law enforcement officials explained, is an attractive stolen good because it is compact and can fetch as much as $25 per 26-ounce (737 g) can. I then read that:

- two men were arrested in connection with an alleged plot to steal formula in Camden, New Jersey;[15]
- four Mexican nationals were arrested for possible involvement in a shoplifting ring that stole at least $30,000 worth of formula from stores in the Oklahoma City area, which is peanuts compared to reported retail formula theft in Texas of $30 million in 2001 and "only" $5 million in 2004 (it is said to be usually shipped to a distribution point, repackaged, re-dated if necessary, re-cased and then distributed on the black market);[16]
- also in Texas, in 2002 investigators linked a gang called MS-13 to a truckload of stolen infant formula, which police suspected at the time was to be sold to support gang operations. A year later a congressional hearing was told that MS-13 members in Texas were suspected of working with fences to steal large amounts of formula, in many cases using shoplifting crews that hit stores in Texas, Oklahoma and Arkansas;[17]
- Albertson's Inc., one of the largest US supermarket chains (2500 stores in 37 states) keeps a few cans of formula on its shelves and directs customers to the service counter if they want more (the executive director of the Infant Formula Council says that formula worth millions of dollars is stolen every year);[18]
- in Tucson, Arizona, where formula can run $75 and up per case, meth users steal and resell it for cash, or sometimes drug dealers will take it to cut drugs;[19]

- a multistate baby-formula investigation called Operation Blackbird led to felony charges against more than 40 suspects;
- authorities seized some $2.7 million in stolen assets, including $1 million worth of formula;
- proceeds from shoplifted formula may be linked to financing international terrorism;[20]
- a Keene, New Hampshire woman was sentenced to one year in jail after stealing nine cans of infant formula (the shoplifting charge was a felony because she had two prior theft convictions, including one for taking seven cartons of cigarettes).[21]

Using "stolen infant formula" as key words, a Google search turns up about 224,000 potential hits. Thus, with ample historical precedent, it appears that infant formula has arrived in considerably more than a nutritional sense. When a commodity assumes an inflated value as a result of market forces like popular perceptions and government intervention, for example large-scale formula giveaways like WIC[22] (see chapter 6), it has the potential of becoming an article of barter and even ill-gotten gain in a parallel economy. As the *Christian Science Monitor* noted, formula is a favorite of theft rings because of the steady demand, high cost, and large profit margins. Formula trading has even arrived on the online auction house eBay, which at the end of March 2006 listed 4,840 items under "infant formula."[23] In contrast, there are reports[24] that eBay has barred the sale of human milk, while since January 2006 a blog on radioball.net has had 100 postings from women seeking to buy or sell milk (see chapter 4).

I think of something as old and vital as salt; its production, distribution, consumption and taxation have been important throughout history whether in the development of societies and states, shaping trade routes across the Sahara or in assembling armies.[25] More recently, duty-free goods – notably tobacco products and alcoholic beverages – are subject to artificially inflated prices due to "sin taxes" and other revenue-generating factors. One observer[26] suggests a common thread to such items insofar as consumption patterns follow the addiction model. It's easy to get hooked and then you've got to have it. Waylaying literally whole truckloads of such high-demand commodities is thus hardly new or unusual. Given a confluence of market conditions, why should infant formula's fortunes – figuratively and literally – be any different?

The use of the funds generated from stolen formula aside, the potentially serious public health impact cannot be overlooked. Where repackaging takes place, it's not unreasonable to assume that a mixture of greed and incompetence play a role in cutting the original full-strength product with all this implies by way of reducing nutritional adequacy and microbiological safety.

April 26, 2005. Riverside, California, USA. Trial and error

John Welsh reports[27] that a 49-year-old emergency-room nurse from Holland, Ingrid Ann Crane, was sentenced, in Riverside, California, to three years in prison on one count of "a lewd act with an infant" for breastfeeding another woman's child while on duty. This is how Welsh describes the case:

- According to co-workers, who filed a complaint, the nurse was engaging in an "unsanitary and disgusting" act.
- According to the judge, who denied probation, it was questionable whether the nurse's remorse was genuine.
- According to the deputy district attorney, Michelle Paradise, the defendant "violated the most vulnerable people of our society."
- According to another mother, who accused the nurse also of breastfeeding her child, she "interfered with a natural loving bond of mother and baby to satisfy her own sick sexual needs."

- According to the law-enforcement officer, Julie Lowry, assigned to investigate, it was the "most bizarre case I've ever encountered" in 17 years' experience.

It seems clear enough that Ingrid Ann Crane has a psycho-affective disorder that needs professional attention, although it's unlikely to be dealt with as long as she's incarcerated. Beyond her emotional problems, however, what concerns me here is the *extreme* hostility of the disapproving language used to describe her actions – "unsanitary," "disgusting," "violated," "sick sexual needs," and "most bizarre" – in conjunction with breastfeeding.

May 9, 2005. London, England. A not so rhetorical question
The world's second biggest-selling English language daily, *The Daily Mail*,[28] put it this way: "We know that breast is best for baby – so why do women in the UK continuously ignore the important health benefits of breastfeeding?"[29] Good question, particularly if you take a look at recent surveys undertaken to coincide with national Breastfeeding Awareness Week:

When the Department of Health published results of its 2004 survey of one thousand women, it noted that the UK had one of the lowest breastfeeding rates in Europe. Almost a third of women in England and Wales never even try to breastfeed, and the rate in Wales among those who do falls to 36% by one month. Younger women in particular are less likely to breastfeed with over 40% of mothers under 24 never trying. The survey also showed that:

- Over a third of women believe that infant formula is very similar to, or the same as, breast milk.
- A fifth of young women aged 16-24 years believe that breastfeeding will ruin the shape of their breasts or body (Gwyneth Paltrow apparently agrees[30]).
- Over two-thirds of women believe that people find breastfeeding in public unacceptable.

- Nearly all women believe that breastfeeding comes naturally to some and not to others.
- Nearly all women believe that some women don't produce enough milk to be able to breastfeed.

Unfortunately, according to the National Childbirth Trust[31] results of a survey undertaken for Breastfeeding Awareness Week 2005 were hardly more encouraging:

- More than 91% of Britons do not know that breastfeeding for just one month has a lasting impact on the first 14 years of life.
- Two thirds are unaware that breastfeeding early in life, even if it is not exclusive, provides protection against infections.
- Only just over half know that the current recommendation is that babies receive breast milk alone for the first six months.
- Almost half do not know that breastfeeding cuts the risk of osteoporosis and ovarian cancer in mothers.

Information from the Avon Longitudinal Study of Parents and Children[32] on the feeding patterns of 11,344 infants at the age of six months found that exclusive breastfeeding declined steadily from 55% in the first month to 31% in the third, and fell to 9.6% in the fourth month due to the introduction of solids (although many mothers were reported to continue to breastfeed their babies).[33]

May 12, 2005. Yangon, Myanmar. Cross-species breastfeeding attempt ends in death[34]

Two Bengal tiger cubs that were breastfed by a Yangon housewife for nearly six weeks have died of dehydration. Three cubs were born at the zoo, but their mother killed one and refused to feed the others. After bottle-feeding failed, the zoo put out a call for breastfeeding mothers. The black-striped orange-brown cubs drew worldwide attention when Hla Htay, a mother of a baby boy, answered the plea for help and fed the cats three times a day. But the cubs – a male and a female born on March 17 – did not take well to human milk. "We did all we could to save them," Dr. Khin Maung Win of the Yangon Zoological Garden told the Myanmar-language Interview Journal. "They were kept in an air-conditioned room, but their livers could not accept human milk." If it won't work in the cubs' direction, should we be surprised that it works so badly in ours?

June 4, 2005. Virginia, USA. Dispatching tyrants
An incident in a Charlottesville, Virginia, fast-food restaurant, The Atomic Burrito, led to public protest – and an apology and policy reversal from restaurant owners – after a member of the staff informed a mother that she couldn't breastfeed her six-month-old on the premises.[35] Atomic Burrito issued the following statement on June 4, 2004:

> *Atomic Burrito strongly supports the rights of mothers and families. Furthermore, Atomic Burrito unconditionally supports the rights of mothers to breastfeed within the restaurant specifically and in public generally. Atomic Burrito does not discriminate on the basis of race, sex, religion, sexual orientation, age or familial status.*

As a result, there is talk about modifying Virginia's right-to-breastfeed law, which currently covers only state property. That's surely an approach consistent with the state's very own official seal. According to the description on the official website,[36] the seal depicts Roman goddess Virtue – her left breast bare – representing the spirit of the Commonwealth of Virginia. She has one foot on Tyranny, who is pictured in a way indicating that struggle has ended in complete victory, followed by the Latin motto, *Sic semper tyrannis*, which I translate freely as: *This* is how we deal with tyrants!

June 7, 2005. New York City. Lactose intolerance

It all began when American television personality and talk-show host (ABC's The View) Barbara Walters said on camera that she felt awkward sitting with her hairdresser on an airplane next to a woman who was breastfeeding. "It made me nervous," Walters said on the May 17 show. "She didn't cover the baby with a blanket. It made us uncomfortable." Co-host Elisabeth Hasselbeck, who was breastfeeding her daughter at the time, said she was "uncomfortable breastfeeding in general" (hardly surprising if you check the first log entry for October 23, 2005). According to one media report,[37] the show's hosts seemed to celebrate the news that Hasselbeck's daughter had her first bottle of formula. Next thing you know nearly 150 angry moms – babies at their breasts – showed up for a feed-in outside ABC's Manhattan studios. Walters said that her airplane anecdote did not reflect her show's stance on the subject. "We're totally supportive if an individual wants to breastfeed."

June 27, 2005. London, England. Barring the unexpected

One of my favorite bits of fantasy research concerns simultaneously having unlimited funds and carte blanche to go into the world's prisons to discover what proportion of the men and women behind bars were themselves ever breastfed as children and, if so, for how long. (Just what do you suppose my null hypothesis[38] would be in a situation like this?) Then, I would seek to correlate breastfeeding rates, past and present, with current national incarceration rates. Even a casual glance at a recent study of comparative imprisonment rates in 211 independent countries and dependent territories suggests an intriguing inverse relationship.[39]

The International Centre for Prison Studies reports that the imprisonment rate in England and Wales is the highest of any major country in Western Europe, 142 out of every 100,000 people. The lowest rates in Europe are found in Scandinavia, with Norway and Sweden (65), Denmark (70) and Finland (71) all well below the international average. Northern Ireland has just 72 but the rate is 132 in Scotland. In Western Europe only Luxembourg, at 144 per 100,000 people, has a higher rate than England and Wales. In Oceania (including Australia and New Zealand) the median rate is 111, whereas it is 117 in Australia and 168 in New Zealand when considered separately. Meanwhile, the USA, with 714 prisoners per 100,000 inhabitants, has remained the country with the highest rate of confinement in the world since 2000 (compared to 116 in Canada). Indeed, of the nine million persons imprisoned worldwide, more than two million (22%) are behind American bars.[40]

August 29, 2005. Portland, Oregon, USA. Frontier justice

The headline reads: "Meth mom sentenced to 18 months in prison."[41] The charge: forcible ingestion of a controlled substance called methamphetamine, which is an extremely addictive synthetic stimulant of the central nervous system sold illegally in pill form, capsules, powder and chunks. Prosecutors hailed this "hallmark case" because it directly holds addicted mothers accountable for the harm they cause their children.

Jennie Thomas of Salem, Oregon, pleaded guilty to a felony: breastfeeding her baby while high on meth. The case arose when she took her nine-month-old son to a hospital because he was not well. Staff noticed that the infant seemed highly agitated and tests showed that he had an extremely high concentration of meth in his system.

Television news anchor Anna Song: "Prosecutors describe this as yet another way of tackling the meth problem by going after mothers who knowingly endanger their children by feeding them drug-tainted breast milk. Nursing is one of the most intimate connections a mother can share with her child, but what if, in doing that, a mother is putting her child at risk?"

A grandmother interviewed: "I think it's really cruel. I don't think that's a good thing at all. To me, endangering a child ... it's one of the worst things you can do."

Sarah Morris, Deputy District Attorney for Marion County: "We as prosecutors have a responsibility to the children in our community to hold parents accountable for the actions against them."

Since Jennie Thomas' husband is also an admitted meth user, both of her children have been removed from her care and placed in state custody while she serves her sentence.

Now, then, what are we to make of a situation like this? For starters, Jennie Thomas has a serious problem of addiction that requires expert treatment, not incarceration. Furthermore, while separation certainly eliminates further risk to her baby through contaminated milk, this is hardly ideal for the short- and longer-term psychosocial health of either mother or child or their future prospects, separately or together. Two wrongs still don't make a right. Unfortunately, with an estimated 2.4 million children in the USA having a parent who is *currently* incarcerated, the situation is hardly unique. Whereas the number of people behind bars has increased five-fold in the last 25 years, the number in on drug charges has increased twelve-fold.[42]

But here is what *really* gets my attention about this story: the parallel between the impact of routine, i.e. non-emergency, formula feeding and the language used here to describe *holding mothers accountable for the harm they cause their children*; feeding described as *one of the most intimate connections a mother can share with her child, but what if, in doing that, a mother is putting her child at risk*; going after *mothers who knowingly endanger their children*; *putting a child at risk* through feeding behavior, which is *one of the worst things you can do*; and having *a responsibility to children in the community to hold parents accountable for the actions against them.*

What about all those moms then who put their kids at risk by pouring infant formula down their throats? How long before they understand the appalling nutritional mediocrity of normalized artificial feeding, this unconscious deviation from the biological norm for the young of our species with its devastating consequences for the health of mothers and children alike throughout the life course?

September 1, 2005. Sydney, Australia. Infant formula as grand metaphor

First I read the headline: "Infant formula makes the taxman whimper."[43] Then I read the article, but no where in it did I find any mention of infant formula or even of feeding babies. Instead, the article described the results of research by the Australian Federal Treasury showing that the tax and welfare changes introduced by Prime Minister John Howard and Treasurer Peter Costello had resulted in a jump in after-tax income by almost a third more than inflation in the first decade (since 1996) of the Howard Government.

Using my powers of deductive reasoning, I then concluded that all 20 of the hypothetical families featured in the Treasury study were failing to breastfeed their children. Furthermore, I determined that these same families were not really making out financially nearly as well as the fat rats in the Howard & Costello Cheese Factory portrayed by the journalist. After all, families that fail to breastfeed their children have to spend quite handsome sums not only on buying a breast-milk substitute but also in contending with the short- and longer-term health fallout, whether for themselves or their children, and this across the entire life course.

Or perhaps I've got it all wrong. Maybe it's nothing more mysterious or complex than a headline writer who saw the words "infant formula" as metaphor, the verbal equivalent of the still-ubiquitous feeding-bottle ideogram in the world's airports; you know, that back-lit black-and-white graphic symbol of a child's feeding-bottle suspended prominently at an angle from terminal ceilings (along with signs indicating where public toilets are located) showing mothers – including, ironically, breastfeeding mothers – where they can go and comfortably feed and otherwise care for their children.

In the mind of the headline writer, then, this was unquestionably how things *really* are child-feeding-wise, at least in Australia. But "infant formula" is not only synonymous with "child feeding;" it appears to have attained the enviable rank of complete societal metaphor covering neatly such key conceptual images as family formation patterns and child-bearing and rearing practices. Yes, that must be it. In fact, I'm sure it is. You see, what convinced me was when I replaced "infant formula" with "breastfeeding" in the headline. Somehow, "Breastfeeding makes the taxman whimper" just doesn't have the same authentic ring.

September 30, 2005. Tel Aviv. How long is "prolonged"?[44]
The report[45] by Mandel and colleagues in Tel Aviv about the fat and energy content of expressed human milk in "prolonged lactation provides as interesting a scientific analysis of the composition of human milk as it does a glimpse at the cultural bias from which the analysis is made. Indeed, the authors' very definition of "prolonged lactation" is at odds with the article's last sentence, which acknowledges the contribution of anthropologist Katherine Dettwyler to our collective understanding of the normal and natural – not the prolonged – duration of breastfeeding for modern humans: 2.5 years at a minimum and about 7 years at a maximum.[46]

The article's last sentence also provides a striking contrast to its first: "The optimal duration of breastfeeding is unknown." Even if *we* don't know yet, from the perspective of child-led weaning it is safe to say that at least the *children* do. Unfortunately, the American Academy of Pediatrics' open-ended recommendation – "Breastfeeding should be continued for at least the first year of life and beyond for as long as mutually desired by mother and child"[47] – has not been cited fully; whereas the World Health Organization's policy – "while breastfeeding continues for up to two years of age or beyond" – has been omitted entirely.[48]

That researchers are only just getting around to investigating human milk's fat and energy content after one year of lactation speaks volumes about breastfeeding's perceived nutritional and psychosocial value for toddlers. It also brings to mind, at the opposite end of the child-feeding spectrum, the widespread belief just a generation ago that human milk was fine but only for babies born at term; that is, until researchers took a look at the milk of mothers who actually delivered preterm and concluded that it was in fact better suited for babies born early.[49]

The statement "Whether continued high saturated fat and cholesterol intake through breastfeeding beyond the first year of life is beneficial in unknown" only serves to reinforce the article's cultural bias. (Why wouldn't it be? After all, it's still milk.) Not so long ago pediatricians considered breast milk to be "low" in iron, at least compared to infant formula. If breast milk is now seen as "high" in saturated fat, to what is it being compared? Milk's fat content varies considerably among species, and even within the same species, for example the kangaroo that routinely produces two milks for different-age offspring. It's time we adopted the perspective that what Mother Nature has provided is the default even as we strive to understand why.

We could also take a cue from the results of Australia's first study of mothers who were breastfeeding children at least two years of age or older (107 mothers aged 21 to 45 years [average 34 years] and 114 children aged 24 to 78 months [average 36 months]). When children were asked about breastfeeding, nearly all said they breastfed because they liked the milk and it made them feel happy or good. They also reported that breast milk tastes "as good as chocolate" and "better than ice cream."[50]

October 10, 2005. Washington, DC, USA. Pushing pacifiers and panning co-sleeping

The American Academy of Pediatrics has revised its SIDS recommendations; they are now in favor of using pacifiers from one month of age and against co-sleeping.[51] The Academy doesn't get a free ride, however; almost immediately the world's foremost mother-to-mother support organization, La Leche League International,[52] and the International Lactation Consultant Association,[53] the Academy of Breastfeeding Medicine[54] and the United States Breastfeeding Committee[55] issued their research-based dissenting responses. The League noted that "the obvious omission of input by the AAP's [own] Section on Breastfeeding may account for the fact that breastfeeding management issues were not taken into consideration." Reaffirming that "the baby who is exclusively breastfed for six months is the appropriate resource model," ILCA noted that "very few of the studies cited in the AAP policy statement defined either exclusivity or duration." The president of the Academy of Breastfeeding Medicine described the statement as "a truly astounding triumph of ethnocentric assumptions over common sense and medical research." Meanwhile, the United States Breastfeeding Committee recommended caution before advising pacifiers for breastfeeding infants even after one month of age. It also emphasized the importance of closeness to one's infant and supported the statement – of the Academy's very own Section on Breastfeeding – that mothers and infants sleep in close proximity.[56]

October 11, 2005. Toronto, Canada. Shutting down the house that Jack built

The North York General Hospital, one of Toronto's largest health facilities, is closing its breastfeeding clinic,[57] which sees more than 1000 mother/baby pairs a year. Run by Dr. Jack Newman together with Dr. Glen Berall and lactation consultant Edith Kernerman, the administration says the hospital cannot afford to house any program that does not directly involve hospital staff. I decided to write a note of support (see also log entries for November 16, 2005 and March 1, 2006):

Honourable George Smitherman
Minister of Health
Ontario, Canada

10 November 2005

Dear Mr. Smitherman,
I would like to add my voice to what I anticipate are the many who have already registered their disappointment and concern at the news of the closure of the internationally known and respected breastfeeding clinic at North York General Hospital. Indeed, I can't help but wonder whether Ontario is aware of the public health pearl in its possession and the positive impact it has had in as diverse environments as France, New Zealand and the USA among others.

During my career in international public health nutrition, with particular emphasis on appropriate infant and young child feeding, I have often been struck by the number of occasions Canadians and non-Canadians alike allude to the important contribution the breastfeeding clinic has made, whether in terms of providing direct support for local mothers, training medical and paramedical personnel, or serving nationally and internationally as a model centre of excellence for others to follow.

Providing mothers and their children the support they need is surely one of the single most cost-effective means of ensuring that breastfeeding – a natural act but a learned behaviour – retains and increases its nutritional and nurturing contribution to the health and well-being of the entire society and across the entire life course. Thus, I dare hope that the competent authorities will carefully reassess what is at stake with the clinic's disappearance.

James Akre
Geneva, Switzerland

October 11, 2005. New Brunswick, Canada. No cover up here[58]

The Irving newspaper group has pulled from store shelves the latest issue of *Here*, a free weekly magazine targeting urban youth, and fired its editor after a close-up photo of a breastfeeding baby appeared on its cover. The photo is an extreme close-up of a tiny suckling baby; the cover promoted a story about World Breastfeeding Week, which began in Canada on October 1, while highlighting the low rates of breastfeeding in New Brunswick.[59] Irving news executives replaced the photo with a cartoon drawing of a woman holding a baby in a blanket. Former *Here* editor Miriam Christensen says she was fired on October 6 after Brunswick News executives recalled the original cover from delivery trucks and stores across the province. She is surprised at her former employer's reaction to the photo and says she didn't think an image of a nursing baby would offend anyone.

Brunswick News vice-president Victor Mlodecki told CBC the original cover was inappropriate for some of the locations that might have distributed it. Freelance journalist Brent MacDonald wrote the story and is angry the photo was pulled. He says the cover was an important part of the piece. "The photo was pulled, the image of a mother breastfeeding her baby, and it really didn't do justice to the story, or the real issue here, that mothers in New Brunswick aren't breastfeeding their babies and babies are being shortchanged." According to a report of the New Brunswick Advisory Council on the Status of Women, 64% of NB mothers who gave birth between 1998 and 2003 breastfed (the national average was 85%) but only 26% breastfed for four months (48% nationally) and 17% past six months (39% nationally).

October 23, 2005. Gordonsville, Virginia, USA.
Introducing the new Bright Beginnings™ spokesmom

I haven't exactly established a dragon-slayer cottage industry, but I occasionally go after a manufacturer or two, especially when they lead so enticingly with their chins as in the following example. I don't expect replies even if one occasionally arrives; my main purpose in writing is to let the Joe Shields of the marketing and promotion fraternity know that they have not yet fooled all the people all the time. Joe never responded. In the context, I'm reminded of the observation that some people use language to express thought, some to conceal thought and others instead of thought. (See also log entries for March 15 and 29, 2006.)

Joe Shields
Director of Public Relations
Bright Beginnings
Gordonsville, Virginia
USA

Dear Mr. Shields,

It was interesting to read the "Meet Elisabeth Hasselbeck" story on the Bright Beginnings website.[60] Indeed, two items in particular caught my attention. First, I was pleased to learn that Elisabeth Hasselbeck is "an active devotee of breast cancer research" and that she continues to support charitable causes including the Susan G. Komen Breast Cancer Foundation. However, I can't help but wonder whether Ms. Hasselbeck has had the opportunity to explore the Foundation's website[61] and especially the section on Risk Factors and Prevention. Perhaps you would be kind enough to draw Ms. Hasselbeck's attention to the section on "Not Breastfeeding," which, with appropriate references to the scientific literature, states:

> *There has been much debate about the effects of breastfeeding on a woman's risk of breast cancer. Although the issue is still under investigation, there is now good evidence that breastfeeding protects against the disease, particularly in premenopausal women.*

In an analysis [62] that combined the results of 47 studies, mothers who breastfed for a total of one year (all children combined) were found to be slightly less likely to develop breast cancer than mothers who had not breastfed. Those who breastfed for a total of two years got about twice the benefit of those who breastfed for a total of one year. Breastfeeding for longer yielded even larger benefits.

Add this reduced risk of breast cancer to the other benefits of breastfeeding – such as fewer childhood infections, fewer sick days used to care for an ill child, a quicker return to pre-pregnancy weight and possibly a lower risk of ovarian cancer – and there are compelling reasons for women to choose to breastfeed their children if the resources are available and they are capable of doing so.

Second, I am pleased to see that Bright Beginnings is striving to ensure that formula-fed babies receive the best possible nutrition by making its infant formula as good as nutritional science permits. However, I have great difficulty accepting the, at best, misleading association of two ideas in the article's final sentence: "For a sensible price, parents can afford a nutritionally complete infant formula with the lipids DHA (docosahexaenoic acid) and ARA (arachidonic acid), two important nutrients found in breast milk that have been proven to aid in babies' brain and eye development." Most assuredly, DHA and ARA – in breast milk – are key to brain and eye development. Nevertheless, according to the latest Cochrane review:[63]

Babies fed with breast milk may have more mature sight skills and a higher IQ (Intelligence Quotient) than babies fed formula. It has been suggested that low levels of long-chain polyunsaturated fatty acids (LCPUFA) found in formula may contribute to lower IQ levels and sight skills. Some formulas are available with added

LCPUFA. This review of trials found that there was not enough evidence to show a long-term benefit of LCPUFA supplementation but that LCPUFA supplementation was safe. More research is needed to assess whether LCPUFA supplementation results in mild improvements in problem solving ability.

This conclusion is consistent with that previously published (The Cochrane Library, Issue 1, 2002):

At present there is little evidence from randomized trials of LCPUFA supplementation to support the hypothesis that LCPUFA supplementation confers a benefit for visual or general development of term infants ... Data from randomized trials do not suggest that LCPUFA supplements influence the growth of term infants.

Obviously, every effort should continue to be made to improve the nutritional quality of infant formula for infants who have to be fed on a breast-milk substitute. At the same time, however, it is important to understand just how inadequate any breast-milk substitute is in the face of so complex a food as breast milk and so multifaceted a feeding method as breastfeeding with their multiple and still-being-discovered ramifications for the health of mothers and children alike throughout the entire life cycle.

James Akre
Geneva, Switzerland

October 23, 2005. Dallas, Texas, USA. All public health recommendations are not created equal: making an exception for breastfeeding
I followed up my letter to Joe Shields with a letter to the Foundation mentioned in the Bright Beginnings press release. No reply here either.

To: The Susan G. Komen Breast Cancer Foundation,
Dallas, Texas

I am writing to say how pleased I am to read the section of your
site on "Not Breastfeeding,"[64] which states:

> *There has been much debate about the effects of
> breastfeeding on a woman's risk of breast cancer.
> Although the issue is still under investigation, there is
> now good evidence that breastfeeding protects against
> the disease, particularly in premenopausal women.*
>
> *Add this reduced risk of breast cancer to the other benefits
> of breastfeeding – such as fewer childhood infections,
> fewer sick days used to care for an ill child, a quicker
> return to pre-pregnancy weight and possibly a lower risk
> of ovarian cancer – and there are compelling reasons
> for women to choose to breastfeed their children **if the
> resources are available and they are capable of doing
> so** (emphasis added).*

However, I do have one suggestion with regard to the last 12
words of this text. Parents are routinely encouraged to protect their
children's lives and well-being by having them vaccinated against
the major childhood diseases and transported in safe car seats, and
by keeping potentially dangerous substances (e.g. medicines and
cleaning products) out of reach. But surely no one would consider
adding a qualifying phrase like "if the resources are available and
they are capable of doing so." There are two points here. The first
is a question of logic – if advice is taken, the health of mothers and
children is protected and the risk of disease, and injury or death,
is lowered, irrespective of resource availability or capability; and,
second it is difficult to see why the nutritional norm for mothers
and babies should be the subject of a qualified endorsement
when every other public-health recommendation is presented in a
straightforward categorical manner.

James Akre
Geneva, Switzerland

October 24, 2005. Madison, Wisconsin, USA. Expanding Mother Nature's market share in America's Dairyland[65]

According to the Wisconsin Milk Marketing Board,[66] agriculture is Wisconsin's leading industry worth an estimated $51.5 billion; dairying, which is larger than both manufacturing and tourism, is the most important segment at $20.6 billion. The Mother's Milk Association of Wisconsin near Madison has received its first donation as the state's first breast milk drop-off center. The collected milk is frozen and shipped to the Ohio Mothers' Milk Bank[67] where it is cultured for bacteria and pasteurized before being returned to Wisconsin. Costing as much as $4 an ounce (29.57 ml) compared to an estimated $1/ounce for infant formula powder,[68] the milk is available with a doctor's prescription. "The beauty of human milk is that it's specific to humans," says Jill Innes, a public health nurse and milk depot volunteer. "So the benefits from one human to another are much greater than from a chemical or a plant or a cow."[69]

October 27, 2005. Dundee, Scotland. The irony and the paradox

Dundee-based Marlyn Glen is a member of the Scottish Parliament and a co-sponsor of the Breastfeeding (Scotland) Act which, since March 2005, protects the right of mothers to breastfeed publicly. Figures released by National Health Service Tayside to Ms. Glen show that, although the number of mothers breastfeeding is rising, fewer than half of all mothers in Dundee are breastfeeding their babies when they are discharged from the hospital.[70] Indeed, rates are far lower than elsewhere in Tayside (the region takes its name from the River Tay and covers 3,000 sq. miles (7,700 sq. km) with a population of 400,000 people). In 1997/1998, only 30% of mothers were breastfeeding at the time of discharge. Though 2003/2004 figures show a rise to

46%, this is still nearly 10% lower than the rate for Tayside as a whole. The real revelation, however, is the rate at six weeks postpartum: only 26.4% of Dundee's babies are being breastfed at this point, the lowest rate in Scotland. (By comparison, just over half of women initiate breastfeeding in Argyll and Clyde, and by six weeks only 32% are still at it.[71])

Oh, the irony and the paradox! It was in Dundee between 1985 and 1989 that Peter Howie and colleagues undertook their history-making study of feeding practices and sickness episodes, especially gastrointestinal disease,[72] among 618 mother-child pairs in the first two years of life. They are considered to be the first researchers to overcome methodological difficulties and demonstrate, once and for all, that even in a middle-class environment in an industrialized country it is, indeed, breastfeeding that makes the significant difference in protecting babies against infection. These results are a beacon in the scientific literature, as is the team's follow-up investigation of the same cohort showing a significantly reduced probability of respiratory illness[73] occurring at any time during childhood for children fed breast milk exclusively for 15 weeks with no solid food. Alas, they appear to be all but forgotten in Dundee, at least as far as today's mothers are concerned.

October 27, 2005. Brattleboro, Vermont, USA. Boo![74]

One Halloween display in Vermont is causing people to look twice, and many can't quite believe what they see. David and Lauren Petrie of Brattleboro decked out their home for Halloween. But it's not pumpkins that are attracting attention. It's "The Witch Lactation Station," a holiday display featuring a breastfeeding witch, complete with a gourd breast and a baby witch doll. Some in town say the display is inappropriate, particularly because their kids are asking questions. Others can see the humor in it, and say it's a great way to raise awareness of breastfeeding. The Petries say they have no plans to take down the display. "We are having fun with it," David Petrie told the

Brattleboro Reformer newspaper. "My four kids were breastfed and we believe it is the best way to feed a child."

October 27 & 29, 2005. Chandler, Arizona, USA. Shoot-out at Chandler Corral

The "controversial breastfeeding issue" that "took center stage at the Chandler City Council meeting"[75] this week concerned a vote to decide whether mothers should be able to breastfeed their children in a public place. The outcome? A unanimous vote cleared the way for mothers to breastfeed "anywhere a mother and child are allowed to be" in Chandler, which becomes only the second city in the country (Philadelphia was first) to enact such a law. Amy Milliron sparked the debate earlier in the year when a lifeguard at a public pool told her that she must breastfeed in the restroom. The City Council also passed a resolution asking the state legislature to follow its lead. Majority Whip Jay Tibshreany said the legislature is hearing from others and is likely to remove breastfeeding from indecent exposure laws during the next session.[76] Thirty-eight US states have laws protecting the right of mothers and their children to breastfeed anywhere they otherwise have a right to be, but Arizona isn't one of them.[77]

November 9, 2005. Charlotte, South Carolina, USA. There's no secret at Victoria's

The refusal last June of a Victoria's Secret sales clerk to let a mother use a dressing room to breastfeed her 10-week-old daughter has morphed into a movement to write breastfeeding rights into South Carolina law. The issue erupted over the summer and for a few days about 25 women staged a "nurse-in," breastfeeding their babies underneath the Victoria's Secret awning. Meanwhile, Charleston breastfeeding counselor Lin Cook asked State Rep. Chip Limehouse (R-Charleston) to introduce legislation permitting a mother to breastfeed her child anywhere she is otherwise authorized to be. "We know from the incredible medical benefits that this is an issue that not only parents need to be concerned with," Cook is quoted as saying. "South Carolina could save $22 million annually in health care costs."[78] The bill was passed by the state House of Representatives on February 14, 2006, and the full Senate vote is imminent. The governor has already vowed to sign the bill into law if adopted.[79]

November 9, 2005. London, England. No offense

It should be an offense to stop mothers breastfeeding in public, Labour's David Kidney (Stafford) urged. He said there were "practical and cultural obstacles," which meant some mothers did not start breastfeeding and others gave up too soon, to the detriment of their children. In a move to give mothers in England and Wales the same protection as mothers in Scotland, on November 8, 2005 David Kidney MP proposed a new parliamentary bill to make it illegal to prevent or harass women breastfeeding in public.[80] Polls show that 84% of the public believe breastfeeding young babies in public should not be a matter of controversy. Yet compared with other European countries, the UK has one of the worst records when it comes to breastfeeding; only one in five babies still breastfeeds at six months of age.[81] His breastfeeding bill gained its first reading but some have described it as standing little chance of becoming law.[82]

November 11, 2005. Whitehouse, New Jersey, USA. Enticing target

According to Health Products Research,[83] pediatricians are the second-biggest promotional target (primary-care doctors are first) of top US drug firms, including GlaxoSmithKline, Abbott Laboratories and Pfizer.[84] The study found that antibiotics known as cephalosporins, analeptics to treat Attention Deficit Disorder, and inhaled nasal steroids were the top three drug types being marketed to pediatricians, followed by other allergy medications, asthma therapies and *infant formula*. According to the research conducted by polling more than 2,300 pediatricians, drug-company representatives made 2.9 million sales calls to pediatricians' offices in the quarter ending August 2005 (compared to 11 million calls for primary-care doctors). Yearly expenditures on promotion, not including samples, totaled $8.6 billion.

November 11, 2005. East Berlin and Kensington, Connecticut, USA. Practicing extremism

To: The Editor, The Berlin Citizen
Subject: Breast feeding the best alternative[85]

The generally accurate, balanced and therefore helpful information that Matteo J. LoPreiato, MD, provides readers is seriously undermined by his article's last two paragraphs. How can feeding in a manner consistent with the biological norm for the young of our species be considered "extremism"? Mothers of "ravenous" breastfed infants should be encouraged to breastfeed longer and more frequently, not to feed formula, which is not only unphysiologic, foreign (and therefore risky as Dr. LoPreiato himself points out) but also nutritionally vastly inferior to breast milk.

Granted, infant formula will sustain life in a pinch, and thank goodness for that. But from a nutritional and developmental standpoint, the abundant scientific literature makes clear artificial feeding's negative implications for both children and mothers – and thus the whole population – across the entire life course. Unfortunately, the common idealized view of infant formula as a perfectly good, albeit second-best (i.e. just below breast milk) source of nourishment for children doesn't allow for even a hint of this disenchanting reality. Infant formula is not the best nutritional alternative to breast milk; it is the least bad.

Two points in the article's last two paragraphs deserve special attention. First, the advice that partial bottle-feeding allows a mother "to make better and more copious milk" is just plain wrong. Without frequent emptying of the mammary gland, milk synthesis will not persist. The more often milk is removed and the more completely it is removed, the more milk the breasts make. The opposite is also true and thus serves as a perfect recipe for "insufficient milk" and permanent recourse to artificial feeding. Second, the egalitarian attitude toward breastfeeding and formula feeding demonstrated in the last paragraph is truly stunning. Babies will most assuredly *not* do well either way, and keeping the baby's best interest in mind always makes breastfeeding the no-brainer default.

James Akre

November 12, 2005. Oshkosh, Wisconsin, USA. Oshkosh B'Gosh[86]

An avalanche of disapproving headlines about tragedy in America's Dairyland whooshes in – 213 articles in the space of 24 hours – and not only from all over the USA but also from around the world, including Canada, England, Germany, India, Qatar and South Africa. They all recount the same terrible tale of a 27-year-old Wisconsin mother with an estimated blood alcohol level of between .15 and .27 percent;[87] she is accused of falling asleep on top of, and suffocating, her four-month-old daughter.

What's my problem? Just this: Only four headlines include information on the mother's highly intoxicated state; 104 headlines focus tendentiously on the fact that she was breastfeeding; and though 105 headlines do not mention breastfeeding, it is amply described in the body of each story.

Here are some examples of the 104 headlines. "Mother crushes infant while breastfeeding in Wisconsin,"[88] "Woman accused of killing baby by falling asleep while breast-feeding,"[89] "Wisconsin mom accused in breast-feeding death,"[90] "Woman accused in baby's breast-feeding death,"[91] "Baby dies while breast feeding,"[92] "Breast-feeding death,"[93] "Breast-feed death horror,"[94] "Breastfeeding baby's death lands sleepy mother in prison,"[95] "Baby dies while breastfeeding. Mother falls asleep on child,"[96] "Infant dies, mom accused of falling asleep while breastfeeding,"[97] "Breastfeeding mom kills baby,"[98] and "Mother accused in breast-feeding death."[99]

Of the only four headlines to mention inebriation, two are from outside the USA: Canada ("Drunk mom crushes tot")[100] and Germany ("Drunk mother accidentally kills child while breastfeeding").[101] Ironically, the latter article is a ten-line summary of a considerably more detailed account from MSNBC under the more provocative – and less informative – title "Mother allegedly kills baby while breastfeeding."[102]

What's my point? Just this: The drunk-as-a-skunk mother was acting irresponsibly in every sense, and this quite irrespective of her feeding mode (indeed, she was already on probation for neglect of the same child at the time of the baby's death). Drinking six double shots while out bowling rendered her physically incapable of caring for her baby daughter, let alone of feeding her in a conscientious manner, whether in or out of bed.

Unless justifiably germane, we expect the mainline media to forgo partisan qualifiers, for example extraneous references to class, ethnicity and national origin, when reporting on most any topic. How, then, can 209 out of 213 headline-writers ignore the obvious proximate cause of this tragedy? How can 104 out of these same 213 headline-writers fix their lurid journalistic gaze, instead, on breastfeeding? Indeed, in the context, of what *possible* relevance is breastfeeding to the tragic death of this four-month-old innocent?

November 15, 2005. Vuniyasi, Fiji. Common sense

A woman who struck her de facto husband with a chopper was spared a jail sentence because she was breastfeeding her six-month-old baby.[103] The court showed leniency to the mother who said she acted to save herself and her baby. She told the court that she was breastfeeding the baby, who would face problems if she went to prison. The magistrate said that since she had pleaded guilty to the offense, the court would give her credit. "Common sense dictates that a jail term will serve no purpose and it will be of disadvantage to the child," the magistrate said. He sentenced her to one year in jail but suspended the sentence for two years.

November 15, 2005. Manchester, England. Better by half
In a review of six studies that examine 3,500 healthy children and 900 with intolerance for gluten, a protein found in wheat, rye and barley, researchers from Central Manchester Children's University Hospital concluded that breastfeeding reduced babies' risk of developing celiac disease by 52%.[104] More research is required, however, since it is not clear whether breastfeeding delays the onset of symptoms or provides permanent protection against the disease.

November 15, 2005. New York City. Having a wail of a time
Ross, a unit of Abbott Laboratories, issued a stinging response to a decision by the National Advertising Review Board that condemned its advertising for Similac Advance infant formula.[105] The NARB said the advertising was "confusing at best" and wrongly gave consumers the impression that Similac boosted babies' immune systems. Ross called the NARB decision – which requires the company stop its Similac advertising – "compromised" because three members of the NARB panel were either missing or arrived late for all or part of the hearings. NARB director Bruce Hopewell responded: "We consider the panel being whole if there's a quorum, at least three out of five. In this case there were four." According to the NARB decision, Abbott had run advertising claiming that "Similac Advance … has been clinically shown to help support the development of a baby's immune system like breast milk … [and results in] immune cell development." The National Advertising Division

of the Council of Better Business Bureaus, a unit of NARB, previously told Abbott to modify that language to avoid giving consumers any impression that Similac is "like" breast milk.

So far, so good; now for the really fun part: a competitor's bow, if not quite a genuflection, at the altar of the sacrosanct level playing field.[106] Ross competitor Mead Johnson appealed to the NARB, hoping to restrict Ross's advertising even further by banning it from using language suggesting that Similac helped babies' immune systems. The NARB ruled that Ross ads were "confusing at best" because it used a disclaimer that "directly contradicts the implied message" that Similac has been "clinically shown" to help support infant immune systems. The disclaimer had said: "The clinical study showed immune cell development. Whether this development provides immune protection like the breastfed infant has not been shown."

November 16, 2005. Toronto, Ontario, Canada. Of mothers, babies and thorns

It's taken more than a month, but the news about the doomed breastfeeding clinic at North York General Hospital (see entry for October 11, 2005) has finally begun to surface in the popular media – first on CBC Radio[107] and then in what many consider Canada's English-language newspaper of record, *The Globe and Mail*.[108] Glenn Berall, chief of pediatrics at North York General said the hospital is closing the clinic so it can expand neonatal programs for its patients. Noting that the kind of service provided by clinic director Dr. Jack Newman can be "carried out in the community," Dr. Berall said his department will bring in a full-time lactation consultant. "It's about concentrating on the patients for whom we have responsibility," he said. "Those who come here to deliver, we need to get them off to the right start." But relocating to a private clinic, Dr. Newman points out, means medical students will miss out on the training he currently provides. "I've been a thorn in the side of many people for many years because I've been outspoken about how poorly we help mothers," he said, referring to what he feels is a lack of support for his work among public health officials. This stands in sharp contrast to the views of many of Dr. Newman's patients, who are battling to keep the clinic open. Meanwhile, the Toronto Star editorializes that "Surely it makes sense ... that a hospital like North York General is the right place for a [breastfeeding] clinic."[109]

November 18, 2005. St. Petersburg, Florida. Time's up

The US Food and Drug Administration is unequivocal: A retailer should not offer for sale any infant formula that has passed its "use by" date, and such formula should be pulled off the retail shelf.[110] In a survey of ten stores conducted the same morning by a local TV news team, four were found to have apparently small quantities of infant formula still on their shelves one, two, four and eleven months past their use-by date.[111] The reported attitudes of two mother-consumers are particularly striking in this regard. "That's a little disturbing to the public," Robyn Cullen said. "Breast milk is supposed to be the best. But if you formula feed, you want it to be as close as possible." Jacqui Nesbitt said that the formula her eight-month-old daughter drinks today sets the tone of her future. "What you do now affects them in the long run. Once she gets in school, the way she'll be able to think, and take in information and everything, the formula, I believe, affects all that." Sure does.[112] Something else I'm sure of: Clearly, these moms view formula as a snugly fitting close second to Mother Nature's Own.

November 19, 2005, on the Web. Default food: Don't leave home without it!

Parents Magazine, which bills itself as "America's #1 family magazine", gives advice for flying with baby.[113] Oops! Somehow they forgot the breast milk.

To: The Editor, Parents Magazine

Thanks for your helpful check-list for air travel with baby. Things are complicated enough for unfettered adults; a 10-month-old in tow can be a real challenge and your 11 points are good reminders about how to reduce stress. Incidentally, I also appreciate seeing the masculine not being used exclusively as the default pronoun. And speaking of default, I wonder if it might be possible for you to alter slightly the second and ninth points on your list to include references to breast milk as the original convenience food for children, for example under **Pack only the essentials.** "Take enough diapers, wipes and, if you're not breastfeeding, formula ..." and under **Bring your own food,** "If you're not breastfeeding, mix infant formula ..."

James Akre
Geneva, Switzerland

November 21, 2005. Norfolk, England. Boyle-White sees red

A young first-time mother only today spoke of her embarrassment and anger at being stopped in June by a policeman because she had been breastfeeding her daughter, who was 28 days old at the time, for five minutes on an outdoor bench while using the baby's buggy with the umbrella up as a shield.[114] Before leaving the town center, a police officer told Margaret Boyle-White that a complaint had been made by an elderly person offended by her breastfeeding. Describing herself as "shocked and upset," she decided to speak out in the hope that "no other young mum will be humiliated in this way." Health visitor Margaret Holtz, who set up Norfolk's first baby café to promote the benefits of breastfeeding, believes that England should follow Scotland's lead by making it an offense for anyone to interfere with a mother feeding milk to children under two years of age[115] whether at the breast or by bottle.

December 2005. Suresnes, France & Bremen, Germany. Whatever the market will bare

The France-based Epica awards, which are in their 19th year, aim "to encourage the highest standard of creativity in European advertising and to help agencies, production houses and photographers to develop their reputations across the continent."[116] Awards are judged by a jury composed of representatives of 32 magazines from 23 countries, including Turkey where the awards ceremony was held, for the second time, in January 2006.

The 2005 winner in the "dairy products" category caused quite a stir in the international breastfeeding community. The image included a full-faced view of a fair-haired baby, who can't be more than 6 to 8 months old, with heavily furrowed brow, squinting eyes, screwed-up nose, pursed lips, jerked-back head, and an evident air of *thorough* "Oh, yuk!" scorn, even disgust. The baby is shown seated (my assumption is that it's all a photomontage) directly opposite an equally fair – but bare and disembodied – right female breast and erect nipple that are the antithesis of those of a typically lactating woman.

Oh, yes, and just to the right of the baby is a large glass of (presumably) cow's milk with the proprietary legend "AMMERLAND DAIRIES" etched across it, followed by "No other." centered just below All this is courtesy of the Bremen-based advertising firm of Wächter & Wächter Worldwide Partners, which have been providing "integrated communication since 1948." Ironically, a quick check of the Ammerland Dairies website[117] appears to confirm that, in fact, the company produces nothing intended for consumption by children under 12 months of age, whether for direct retail or wholesale marketing purposes (a request to the company for confirmation went unanswered).

Recalling the standard injunction against whole cow's milk before a child's first birthday, and also bearing in mind that breast milk remains the liquid refreshment of choice for a one-year-old child, there are at least three other dimensions to this

Franco-German travesty in the sociocultural context. First, this is a prime example of the first rule of advertising – Be noticed at all cost! Second, the ad's creators would doubtless argue that their brainchild was merely being cute; the implied rejection of the human in favor of the bovine shouldn't be taken literally (Hey, lighten up; we're just using a figure of speech!). And third, having achieved the approval of their peers by winning a prestigious prize, the creators would no doubt be truly puzzled – even totally clueless – to be rebuked for so unceremoniously smacking Mother Nature across the chops this way. Unfortunately, many in the viewing public would be equally clueless. Question: What's wrong with this picture? Answer: Nothing.

December 2, 2005. New Plymouth, New Zealand. Ladies' lounge litigant

Amy Barton has twice been told not to breastfeed in the lounge area of a District Council-owned restroom and to use the designated area instead – a small room off the toilets.[118] She was told that people waiting for the bus – on the other side of the road – might be able to see her. Barton has complained to the Council and is also thinking of going to the Human Rights Commission. Ironically, many New Plymouth cafes and other business are reported to have adopted the Baby Friendly policy of providing a supportive breastfeeding environment. Council facilities manager Steve Crowe said that women who wanted to would now be permitted to breastfeed in the lounge, although signs directing them to the designated area would remain. Saying that he believed the rule against using the lounge for breastfeeding was a hangover from a bygone era, Crowe referred to a Council survey showing that a number of women didn't want to see breastfeeding in the lounge. A Taranaki Daily News spot survey of ten women using the restroom showed that none had a problem with mothers breastfeeding in the lounge.

December 2, 2005. San Ysidro, California, USA. Bordering on harassment

Zayra Cano, age 18, whose legal residence is in San Ysidro, has filed a complaint against the US Customs and Border Protection Service.[119] Cano told the San Diego Union-Tribune that she was in the back seat breastfeeding when she and her parents, fiancé and baby arrived at the border on their return from Tijuana, Mexico. An agent accused her of child smuggling and told her to produce milk. A service spokeswoman told the newspaper the incident is being investigated. Inspectors who suspect a baby's identity are supposed to ask for a birth certificate – which Cano said she supplied – and can demand a secondary inspection. And what if she had been bottle-feeding?

December 2, 2005. Paris, France. Emotion in the consumer-decision driver seat

According to Professor Lynn Frewer of the University of Wageningen in the Netherlands, unless the food industry accepts that emotional connections drive consumer decisions about what is and what is not acceptable, full public confidence will be hard to restore.[120] This was all the more topical an observation given the recent withdrawal of infant formula in Italy, France, Greece, Portugal and Spain because of packaging ink migrating into the product[121] (see chapter 7). "Consumers do not like surprises – like finding ink in their baby milk formula," said Olivier Mignot from Nestlé's research center in Switzerland at the food safety seminar. "We therefore need to build safety into the design of the food and anticipate news risks. Meanwhile, the European Food Safety Authority has said that it considers the chemical ITX used in packaging inks, though "undesirable," to be of "low health concern."[122] It said young children were likely to have greater exposure to ITX as a large number of beverages consumed by children were likely to be packed in small-volume containers whose levels of ITX were found to be relatively higher than in bigger cartons. The statement followed a detailed analysis by the

Authority's scientific panel on food additives of four types of milk-based products, including infant formula.

December 3, 2005. Ashton-in-Makerfield, England. Actress comes out for breastfeeding

Movie actress Kate Hudson, 26, "admits she breastfed her son in front of the director" when filming 'The Skeleton Key.'[123] The actress, who gave birth to her son 22 months ago, told Britain's *Ok!* magazine: "It was a funny when I was breastfeeding because every three hours I'd go to the trailer to breastfeed or pump. It became a joke in the end … it got to the point where I didn't want to go back to the trailer so I'd just bring the baby out and I'd sit and talk to the director and just breastfeed him while chatting."

December 5, 2005. Beijing, China. Formula for disaster (1)

Two Chinese factory officials have been jailed for producing a baby formula so low in nutrition that it killed one baby girl and left others dangerously malnourished, state media reported.[124] The girl was one of more than 200 infants who suffered malnutrition after drinking phony formula in Anhul, where investigators found the sale of counterfeit milk powder was widespread. At least 12 babies died from drinking other brands of fake formula. The factory produced the shoddy milk powder between 2002 and 2004, the report said. Some 240,000 packages have since been confiscated. China suffers from rampant counterfeiting of food and medicines, but the milk powder cases caused a national uproar after pictures of malnourished infants appeared on television and in newspapers. More than 130 merchants, milk producers and officials were arrested, and several local commerce officials and merchants have already been imprisoned (see also chapter 7 and log entry for February 17, 2006).

January 11, 2006. Ontario, Canada. Shall I compare thee to a … football league?!

Janet (Wardrobe Malfunction) Jackson,[125] where are you when we need you? In a contact sport – Canadian football – notorious for its commentators' overblown rhetoric, what are we to make of sportswriter Mike Camerlengo's choice of analogy when providing his winning-team forecast for 2006?[126] First, his opening paragraph: "The NFC [Northern Football Conference] is *like public breastfeeding* to me; I don't want to watch it, but mainly because there is nothing else going on, I become intrigued. It is ugly and somewhat unnatural, but I want to see what happens in the end." Mike then proceeds to provide his season picks before closing this way: "Those picks are about as solid as the contents of infants (sic) diaper [especially those who are breastfed?] but as of now, that's all I got for you. Maybe these NFC games will be filled with high-placed play and become an offensive shootout. If that's the case, that *breastfeeding mother* just might turn out to be Pamela Anderson instead of the usual Star Jones [lawyer, former prosecutor, and American television personality, who had a self-described 'boob lift'[127] after losing 150 lbs. (68 kg)]." Is the sportswriter's copy an example of art imitating life imitating art – or the reverse?

January 14, 2006. On the Internet. Breast cancer site needs reconstructing

The press release[128] – *Breast cancer site to remain 'under construction': by its readers* – describes a new website called Breast Cancer Information,[129] which will "change daily to reflect readers' needs." Webmaster Charlie (*Nomen est omen*) Allnut of Allnut Enterprises[130] assures visitors that the site welcomes their specific questions, which will be answered "as quickly as possible." So I wrote Charlie on January 15, 2006, to ask him about the site's entry called "Breast cancer for beginners," which states: "There are many myths attached to breast cancer … it was a popular belief earlier that breast-feeding decreases one's risk of the cancer but it has now been found to be untrue."[131] I asked Charlie if he could let me have the relevant references to the scientific literature about breastfeeding's ineffectiveness in terms of lowering the risk of breast cancer. I'm still waiting for Charlie's reply.

January 15, 2006. Salt Lake City, Utah, USA. Apparent pothead parent pardoned

The Utah Court of Appeals has reversed a district court judge's decision to bind over a woman for trial on a third-degree felony charge of child endangerment for breastfeeding her child after smoking marijuana.[132] The court said child welfare officials did not support their claim that the drug entered breast milk, or in what quantities, by any scientific testimony or study. The mother allegedly admitted that she had smoked marijuana once in December 2003 and a second time in January 2004. "The question of whether marijuana was actually present in [the mother's] breast milk when she nursed appears to be of sufficient scientific complexity as to be 'beyond the realm of common experience'," the ruling said.

January 16, 2006. McMinnville, Tennessee, USA. Pump brake

Angela Smith claims in a suit she has filed that she followed unwritten procedures given by supervisors when she returned from maternity leave by notifying her supervisors when she was leaving her work area to use a breast-milk pump during her two 15-minute breaks per 12-hour shift.[133] She was fired because of her alleged failure to follow hospital guidelines, which she noted that other employees, leaving to take smoke breaks outdoors, do not follow.

February 17, 2006. Beijing, China. Formula for disaster (2)

China ordered the recall of baby formula with dangerously low nutritional value two years after dozens of babies died drinking counterfeit formula. The recall was ordered by the Health Ministry after inspectors discovered the inferior formula in rural markets, the official Xinhua News Agency said. In 2004 dozens of babies in eastern China died of malnutrition after being fed counterfeit formula (see also chapter 7 and log entry for December 5, 2005). Merchants distributing that formula were sentenced to prison.[134]

February 18, 2006. Washington, DC. Holy cow

Luiza Ch. Savage is the Washington bureau chief for Maclean's, the popular Canadian weekly newsmagazine that celebrated its centennial in 2005. She contributed a remarkable first-person account about skipping the breastfeeding class during her "typical yuppie pregnancy" with the eye-catching title/lead combination: "Oh baby. My life as a dairy cow. Why would I pay someone to show me how to stick a boob in a baby's mouth? How hard could nursing be?"[135] Well, very hard as things turned out; and this was my reaction.

To: The Editor, Maclean's
Subject: Oh baby. My life as a dairy cow

In 40 years of observing the child-feeding horizon, I've seen a lot of irredeemably vitriolic breastfeeding blather – unfortunately, usually written by women – but Ms. Savage's [account] nearly creates a category of its own. It's also a good example of the adage about a little bit of information being a dangerous thing. Her anger is directed everywhere except where it belongs: with a society that sold her a shoddy, incomplete bill of goods, that taught her "breast is best" without providing her the information and the skill base to act appropriately on that teaching.

I said "irredeemably" but that's not quite true. The writer finally interrupts her rant in the last three paragraphs to describe her positive experience with the "breast guru of Washington." But by the time I got there I was so worn out that it almost didn't matter, a little like recalling wistfully that the Red Cross and the Geneva Conventions got their start at the 1859 Battle of Solferino where many thousands were butchered.

Is it the flawed perception that breastfeeding is so utterly intuitive that leads many observers to assume a no-instructions-required attitude in this regard, and then to be surprised that it's "so difficult"? This remarkably common premise – and sure-fire recipe for disappointment and failure – is especially ironic if you consider how lacking in positive breastfeeding role models so much of popular culture is today.

What's the antidote? In the short term, a knowledgeable but dispassionately written rebuttal might help a little. But in the longer term our best hope is to transform culture and society as a whole since it is they that are responsible for the complex value system that results in more – or variously less – breastfeeding by the mothers and children in their midst.

James Akre
Geneva, Switzerland

March 1, 2006. Melbourne, Australia. All balled up

A full two weeks before the start of the XVIII Commonwealth Games (March 15-26, 2006) media accounts surfaced about the pressure on top netballer medal hope Janine Illitch to stop breastfeeding her six-month-old baby before the Games began.[136] For the 10 days the dual gold medalist was set to reside in the Games village, she was determined to go on breastfeeding. "I'm sure there's a way to do it," she said. "I feel very strongly that I want to continue breastfeeding. It's my right. I'm just an ordinary woman who likes feeding and I want it to be my decision when I stop." But coach Norma Plummer thought differently. "We don't have our own bedrooms and facilities. There are also other people to consider. There's not a lot of room and the players might need their rest and she is in there expressing." Plummer said Netball Australia supported Illitch, paying for her mum, Helen, to fly to Canberra to help look after the baby; but she also said that medical staff were concerned the super-fit Illitch would lose weight if she continued to breastfeed. However, Netball Australia chief executive Lindsay Cane said that coaches (including Plummer), support staff and players were united in supporting Illitch.[137]

March 1, 2006. Toronto, Canada. Opening back up the house that Jack built

The Canadian College of Naturopathic Medicine announced that it is welcoming the Newman Breastfeeding Clinic and Institute to its new location. Jack Newman, clinic founder and pediatrician, started the first hospital-based breastfeeding clinic in Canada in 1984. The new location at the College provides an opportunity for it to become an educational institution with teaching and training for midwives, physicians and other health professionals. North York General Hospital had shut down the clinic in December 2005, citing shortage of space and resources (see log entries October 11 and November 16, 2005).

March 15, 2006. Gordonsville, Virginia, USA. Tell 'em Joe sent you!

Having said hello to Bright Beginnings™, let's welcome New Ultra Bright Beginnings™ DHA-supplemented infant formula. After reminding us that Elisabeth Hasselbeck is still company "spokesmom" – but hey, didn't she breastfeed her daughter?! (see log entry for June 7, 2005) – company contact Joe Shields reports on a "recent survey of new mothers"[138] (minus any indication of numbers or methodology used). Results, he says, were released in conjunction with the launch of Ultra Bright Beginnings infant formula, which is described as offering the highest levels of DHA among national formula brands. Although 93% of new moms have heard of DHA and correctly identified it as a nutrient, 97% do not know the daily recommended level of DHA for infants. Fortunately, director of public relations Joe Shields is there to fill the information void and pinpoint the source of moms' ignorance: Doctors aren't talking about DHA! ("Approximately 73% of new moms rely on their doctor's recommendation for formula choices; however, 83% of respondents indicated that their doctors did not talk to them about DHA.") Unfortunately, as noted earlier (see log entry for October 23, 2005), DHA found naturally in breast milk and added to infant formula just doesn't seem to behave the same way.

March 29, 2006. Gordonsville, Virginia, USA. The method to their madness.

Joe Shields and the gang at PBM Products have obviously been busy. Now it's time for "Parent's Choice ORGANIC Infant Formula with a Blend of Lipids DHA and ARA,"[139] which "is produced without using pesticides (sic), added (sic) growth hormones, or antibiotics." And of course they're only responding to consumer demand, attributing their success to "a continuing dialogue with our customer base and our unique ability to understand and meet evolving needs," says Paul Manning, PBM CEO. This time details are provided concerning "a recent organic survey of 322 new moms" (a nationally representative sample of mothers of children 0-12 months with a +/-3% margin of error).

But what really gets my attention is the evolution in how the PBM press release describes DHA and ARA this time around compared to earlier company declarations – "fatty acids found naturally in mother's milk *associated with* [emphasis added] brain and eye development."[140] Here are three earlier formulations:

- "two important nutrients found in breast milk *that have been proven* [emphasis added] to aid in babies' brain and eye development" (see log entry October 23, 2005);
- "… formula with DHA, an ingredient *believed to stimulate* [emphasis added] brain and retina development;"[141]
- "nutrients naturally found in breast milk *that are essential* [emphasis added] for babies' mental and visual development."[142]

But of course, no matter how much wiggle-room slack PBM cuts itself in this connection, the fact remains that the highly respected Cochrane Collaboration[143] recently concluded, yet again, that "the review of trials found that there was not enough evidence to show a long-term benefit of LCPUFA supplementation [in infant formula]"[144] (see log entry October 23, 2005).

References

1. Kelly W. Zeroing in on those polluters: We have met the enemy and he is us. The Best of Pogo. Mrs. Walt Kelly and Bill Couch Jr. (eds.), Simon & Schuster, 1982 http://www.igopogo.com/final_authority.htm.

2. Australian police bar Aboriginal women from topless dancing, Channel NewsAsia, February 27, 2004 http://www.channelnewsasia.com/stories/australasia/view/72995/1/.html.

3. Topless dancers greet prince. cnn.com, March 2, 2005 http://www.cnn.com/2005/WORLD/asiapcf/03/02/charles.outback/.

4. Ferragamo: Mamma mia! *Daily News*, Daily Dish, May 11, 2004. http://www.nydailynews.com/news/gossip/story/192096p-166047c.html.

5. Mary Jane is a term in the USA for strap shoes. See: http://en.wikipedia.org/wiki/Mary_Jane_(shoe).

6. No nipples, please, we're British as breastfeeding film is censored. *The Herald*, London, May 21, 2004.

7. Nipple causes ripple in the land that invented Page 3 girls. *The Sydney Morning Herald*, May 24, 2004. Wikipedia reports that a Page Three girl is a woman who models for topless photographs published in the UK tabloid *The Sun* http://en.wikipedia.org/wiki/Page_3_girl.

8. Teutsch D. Church playgroup bans breastfeeding mothers. *The Sydney Morning Herald*, June 13, 2004 http://www.smh.com.au/articles/2004/06/12/1086749944208.html?oneclick=true.

9. Women's Health Action Trust, Newmarket, Auckland, New Zealand http://www.womens-health.org.nz/.

10. Richard Prosser, personal communication, November 10, 2005.

11. American Academy of Pediatrics, Section on Breastfeeding. Breastfeeding and the Use of Human Milk, *Pediatrics*, 2005, 115:496-506.

12. Petition 2002/139 of Elizabeth Weatherly and 8,992 others. New Zealand House of Representatives, Report of the Health Committee http://www.clerk.parliament.govt.nz/Content/SelectCommitteeReports/hepet02139.pdf.

13. Human Rights Commission, News & Issues. More to do to promote breastfeeding rights. Wellington, April 13, 2005 http://www.hrc.co.nz/home/hrc/newsandissues/promotingbreastfeedingrights.php.

14. Cigarettes, formula looted from market. *The News & Observer*, Raleigh, NC, April 24, 2005.

15. McCullen S. Infant formula theft is investigated by police. *Bridgeton News*, Bridgeton, NJ, May 5, 2005.

16. Associated Press. Four people suspected in baby formula theft ring. Oklahoma City, Oklahoma, May 28, 2005.

17. War M. New breed of street gang spreads through Texas, U.S. MS-13 viewed as terrorists by feds. *American-Statesman*, Austin (Texas), January 22, 2006.

18. Rubinkam M. Powdered baby formula goes behind counter. Bethlehem, PA, Associated Press, June 3, 2005 http://www.msnbc.msn.com/id/8088953/.

19. Perla N. Stores put powdered baby formula under lock & key. KVOA TV, Tucson, June 8, 2005 http://www.kvoa.com/Global/story.asp?S=3446645.

20. Clayton M. Is black-market baby formula financing terror? *The Christian Science Monitor*, Boston, MA, June 29, 2005 http://www.csmonitor.com/2005/0629/p01s01-usju.html.

21. Associated Press. Woman sentenced to a year in jail after stealing infant formula. Boston.com, November 7, 2005.

22. The Special Supplemental Nutrition Program for Women, Infants and Children (WIC) serves to safeguard the health of low-income women, infants and children up to age five who are at nutritional risk by providing nutritious foods supplement diets, information on healthy eating, and referrals to health care http://www.fns.usda.gov/wic/aboutwic/default.htm.

23. http://baby.listings.ebay.com/Feeding_Baby-Formula_W0QQsacatZ37626QQsocmdZListingItemList

24. Austin M. Sides clash over putting price on mothers' milk. *Denver Post*, March 26, 2006.

25. Salary derives from the Greek root sal-, meaning salt, and the Latin salarium, a payment made in salt. In Rome the soldier's pay was originally salt. In medieval times salt was a valuable barter commodity. This is also the source of the proverb "to be worth one's salt". See: http://en.wikipedia.org/wiki/Salary.

26. Professor George Kent, Department of Political Science, University of Hawai'i, personal communication.

27. Welsh J. Nurse sentenced to prison in breast-feeding case. *The Press-Enterprise*, April 26, 2005.

28. With a circulation of about 2,343,000 (2002) according to Wikipedia http://en.wikipedia.org/wiki/Newspaper_circulation.

29. Breastfeeding Awareness Week 2005, *Daily Mail*, May 9, 2005.

30. WEBINDIA123.COM. Gwyneth Paltrow's breast feeding blues! December 26, 2005. Excerpt: "Paltrow, who has a 19-month-old daughter, and is reportedly pregnant again, blames breastfeeding for changing her shape for the worse, and now regards having surgery as a necessity rather than an indulgence."

31. The National Childbirth Trust, Alexandra House, Oldham Terrace, Acton, London W3 6NH, England http://www.nct.org.uk/.

32. The Avon Longitudinal Study http://www.alspac.bristol.ac.uk/welcome/index.shtml, based at the University of Bristol, is aimed at identifying ways in which to optimize the health and development of children.

33. 90% of mums stop breastfeeding exclusively after 4 months, UK. Medical News TODAY, March 25, 2006.

34. Breast-fed tiger cubs die of dehydration. MSNBC, May 12, 2005 http://www.msnbc.msn.com/id/7824645/.

35. Seen around town: breast feeding, protests and The Atomic Burrito, June 2004 http://george.loper.org/~george/trends/2004/Jun/987.html.

36. Virginia Symbols, Great Seal http://www.shgresources.com/va/symbols/seal/.

37. Meyer K. Lactose Intolerant! *New York Daily News*, June 7, 2005.

38. In statistics, a null hypothesis is a hypothesis that is presumed true until statistical evidence in the form of a hypothesis test indicates otherwise. See: http://en.wikipedia.org/wiki/Null_hypothesis.

39. King's College London, International Centre for Prison Studies. World Prison Population List (sixth edition), June 2005, http://www.kcl.ac.uk/depsta/rel/icps/world-prison-population-list-2005.pdf.

40. Readers please note: As tempting as it might be to nod knowingly and say "Of course", I've described a correlation, not a cause-effect relationship.

41. Meth mom sentenced to 18 months in prison. Anna Song and KATU 2 News Web staff, Portland, Oregon, August 29, 2005.

42. Bernstein N. All alone in the world: children of the incarcerated. New York, The New Press, 2005.

43. Infant formula makes the taxman whimper. John Garnaut, *The Sydney Morning Herald*, September 1, 2005.

44. Akre J. How long is "prolonged"? Post-publication Peer Review, *Pediatrics*, September 30, 2005, http://pediatrics.aappublications.org/cgi/eletters/116/3/e432.

45. Mandel D. Fat and Energy Content of Expressed Human Breast Milk in Prolonged lactation. *Pediatrics* 2005; 116; e432-e435 http://pediatrics.aappublications.org/cgi/content/full/116/3/e432.

46. Dettwyler K. When to wean: biological versus cultural perspectives. *Clinical Obstetrics and Gynecology* 2004;47:712-723.

47. American Academy of Pediatrics. Breastfeeding and the Use of Human Milk. *Pediatrics* 2005; 115-506 http://www.breastfeedingtaskforla.org/resources/AAP%202005%20Breastfeeding%20and%20the%20Use%20of%20Human%20Milk.pdf.

48. Global Strategy for Infant and Young Child Feeding. Geneva, World Health Organization, 2003 http://www.who.int/nut/documents/gs_infant_feeding_text_eng.pdf

49. Lemons JA et al. Differences in the composition of preterm and term milk during early lactation. *Pediatric Research* 1982;16:113-117.
50. Gribble K. Breastfeeding into toddlerhood and beyond: the experience of mothers and children. Breastfeeding the Natural State. Australian Breastfeeding Association International Conference, Hobart, September 28-30, 2005.
51. AAP Revises SIDS Prevention Recommendations, October 10, 2005 http://www.aap.org/ncepr/sids.htm.
52. La Leche League Responds to AAP policy statement on Sudden Infant Death Syndrome, October 14, 2005, http://www.lalecheleague.org/Release/sids.html.
53. ILCA responds to policy statement on AAP Task Force on SIDS. International Lactation Consultant Association http://www.ilca.org/news/SIDSstatementresponse.php.
54. Breastfeeding is Associated with a Lower Risk of SIDS According to The Academy of Breastfeeding Medicine, October 14, 2005, http://www.bfmed.org/documents/SIDS-Bedsharing.doc.
55. United States Breastfeeding Committee, October 17, 2005. Mixed Credibility of the Revised AAP SIDS Prevention Recommendations http://www.usbreastfeeding.org/News-and-Events/USBC-SIDS-PR-10-17-2005.pdf.
56. 2005 AAP Policy Statement on Breastfeeding and the Use of Human Milk, *Pediatrics* 2005; 115; 496-506 http://www.breastfeedingtaskforla.org/resources/AAP%202005%20Breastfeeding%20and%20the%20Use%20of%20Human%20Milk.pdf.
57. Infant Feeding Action Coalition, Toronto breastfeeding clinic faces closure, October 11, 2005 http://www.infactcanada.ca/Action_Alert_Oct1105_1.htm.
58. CBC News, October 11, 2005. Irving news pulls breastfeeding cover, fires editor. cbc.ca New Brunswick http://nb.cbc.ca/regional/servlet/View?filename=nb_breastpaper11102005.
59. MacDonald B. *Here*, Vol. 6, Issue 40, October 6-13, 2005. Breast Assured. A mother and the experts get the facts off their chests http://www.herenb.com/saintjohn/issues/0640/cover.html.
60. Bright Beginnings™. "To a new mom, everything matters."™ http://www.brightbeginnings.com/customer/elisabeth-hasselbeck-spokesmom.asp.
61. http://www.komen.org/intradoc-cgi/idc_cgi_isapi.dll?IdcService=SS_GET_PAGE&nodeId=1000
62. Collaborative Group on Hormonal Factors in Breastfeeding. Breast cancer and breastfeeding: collaborative reanalysis of individual data from 47 epidemiological studies in 30 countries, including 50302 women with breast cancer and 96973 women without the disease. *Lancet*, 2002, 360(9328)203-10.

63. Simmer K. Longchain polyunsaturated fatty acid supplementation in infants born at term. *The Cochrane Database of Systematic Reviews* 2005 Issue 3 http://www.cochrane.org/reviews/en/ab000376.html.

64. http://www.komen.org/intradoc-cgi/idc_cgi_isapi.dll?IdcService=SS_GET_PAGE&nodeId=1000.

65. "America's Dairyland" is the easily recognized slogan on Wisconsin's license plates. Among the state's credentials for the title are national leadership in dairy production and a history of being among the leaders in most milk products since shortly after the first cheese factory was opened in the state in 1864. Encyclopaedia Britannica online http://www.britannica.com/ebi/article-9277774.

66. Wisconsin Milk Marketing Board http://www.wisdairy.com/.

67. Mothers' Milk Bank of Ohio http://dev2-ohiohealth.vianow.com/services/womenshealth/maternity/classesandsupport/breastfeeding/mothersmilkbank.htm

68. Tam J. Baby formula powder "disappearing." KLTV, Tyler, Longview, Jacksonville TX, June 26, 2005.

69. Thomas J. Breast milk depot to feed Wisconsin babies. Madison, *The Daily Cardinal*, November 4, 2005.

70. Morkis, S. Dundee mums less likely to breastfeed. *Evening Telegraph and Post*, Dundee, Scotland, October 28, 2005, http://www.eveningtelegraph.co.uk/output/2005/10/27/story7682469t0.shtm.

71. Breast start. *Greenock Telegraph*, Greenock, May 26, 2005.

72. Howie PW et al. Protective effect of breast feeding against infection. *British Medical Journal*, 1990, 300:11-16.

73. Wilson AC et al. Relation of infant diet to childhood health: seven year follow up of cohort of children in Dundee infant feeding study. *British Medical Journal*, 1998, 316:21-25.

74. CBS4 Boston, Breastfeeding Witch Causing Stir in Vermont, October 28, 2005 http://cbs4boston.com/seenon/local_story_300112352.html.

75. Mother who incited breastfeeding debate speaks out, October 29, 2005. CBS 5 News, kpho.com. http://www.kpho.com/Global/story.asp?S=4038131&nav=23Ku.

76. Jensen E. Nursing moms become advocates. *The Arizona Republic*, October 28, 2005.

77. Breastfeeding and the Law. La Leche League International http://www.lalecheleague.org/LawMain.html and the National Conference of State Legislatures, 50 State Summary of Breastfeeding Laws http://www.ncsl.org/programs/health/breast50.htm.

78. Eichel H. Breast-feeding advocates to rally. Lingerie store incident prompts call to make public nursing legal. *The Charlotte Observer*, November 9, 2005.

79. In the legislature. *The Post and Courier*, Charleston, South Carolina, March 29, 2006.

80. Westminster debates public breastfeeding bill. UNICEF UK Baby Friendly Initiative, November 29, 2005.

81. Thompson J. Do you find breastfeeding offensive? *The Independent* (London), December 18, 2005.

82. *The Guardian* (London). Yesterday in Parliament, November 9, 2005.

83. http://www.hprintl.com/.

84. Gilcrest L. Pediatricians 2nd biggest drug ad target. United Press International, November 11, 2005.

85. LoPreiato MJ. *The Berlin Citizen*, East Berlin, Connecticut. Breast feeding the best alternative, November 11, 2005 http://www.theberlincitizen.com/articles/2005/11/10/local_news/news10.txt.

86. For readers unfamiliar with US retail clothing history and folklore, OshKosh B'Gosh, Inc. was founded in Oshkosh, Wisconsin in 1895 as a manufacturer of adult work wear. It is today a global marketer of children's clothing and accessories.

87. Allowing for variations by sex and weight, at a blood alcohol level of .30 ml of alcohol per 100 ml of blood, or milligrams percent, many subjects lose consciousness, while at .40 most lose consciousness and some die.

88. KUTV, Salt Lake City, Utah, November 12, 2005.

89. *Mumbai Mirror*, Mumbai, India, November 13, 2005.

90. *Herald News Daily*, November 12, 2005.

91. *Houston Chronicle*, November 13, 2005.

92. CBS NEWS, cbs.com, November 12, 2005.

93. WXOW TV, wxoy.com, LaCrosse, Wisconsin, November 12, 2005.

94. *New York Post*, Online Edition, November 13, 2005.

95. *London Free Press*, London, Ontario, November 13, 2005.

96. Associated Press, November 12, 2005.

97. WBIR-TV, wbir.com, Knoxville, Tennessee, November 12, 2005.

98. News24.com, Cape Town, November 12, 2005.

99. *Gulf Times Newspaper*, Doha, Qatar, November 13, 2005.

100. *Ottawa Sun*, November 13, 2005.

101. ShortNews.com, November 13, 2005.

102. MSNBC.com, November 12, 2005.

103. *Fiji Times*, November 15, 2005.

104. United Press International, London. Breast milk halves gluten intolerance risk, November 15, 2005.

105. Brandweek.com, Abbott Labs wails about ruling on baby formula ads, November 15, 2005.

106. A marketing environment in which all companies must play by the same rules and are thereby supposedly given an equal opportunity to compete.

107. Metro Morning, CBC Toronto, November 15, 2005.

108. Stuffco J. A mother's hero, a 'thorn' in hospital's side. *The Globe and Mail*, Toronto, November 16, 2005, and Stuffco J. Petition to save breastfeeding clinic fails to reverse decision on closing it. *The Globe and Mail*, Toronto, November 18, 2005.

109. Nursing mothers deserve best care (editorial). *Toronto Star*, November 18, 2005.

110. USDA, Notice to retailers: Sale of infant formula past the "use by" date, December 22, 1999.

111. WTSP TV, Tampa/St. Petersburg, 10 News Extra: Expired infant formula on store shelves, November 18, 2005.

112. See chapter 10 for references to the implications of infant-feeding mode for cognitive development.

113. Bender M. Have baby, will travel. *Parents Magazine*, November 19, 2005.

114. Wigg C. Breastfeeding mum's upset at complaint. *Eastern Daily Press*, November 21, 2005.

115. BBC News, UK Edition. Breastfeeding bill gains approval, November 18, 2004.

116. epica: europe's premier creative awards http://www.epica-awards.org/epica/2005/winners/preview-print.htm.

117. Molkerei Ammerland (in German only) http://www.molkerei-ammerland.de/index.php.

118. Hulbert J. Restroom rules anger breastfeeding mother. Wellington, *Taranaki Daily News*, December 2, 2005.

119. Mom says border agent made her lactate. NewsTrack, United Press International, December 2, 2005.

120. Fletcher A. Consumer connection vital to restoring faith in food industry. Food Navigator.com/Europe, December 2, 2005.

121. Swiss Info / Swiss Radio International. Nestlé forced to withdraw baby milk, November 23, 2005.

122. ITX considered 'low health concern' by EU food authority. TODAYonline.com, December 10, 2005.

123. Femalefirst.co.uk Kate Hudson's public breast-feeding, December 3, 2005.

124. Chinese manufacturers jailed over deadly formula. Associated Press. CTV Television, Scarborough, Ontario, December 5, 2005.

125. Olbermann K. Janet Jackson's wardrobe malfunction. Full coverage of the un-coverage. MSNBC, February 3, 2004 http://www.msnbc.msn.com/id/4147857/. You don't need to be a fan of American football to have heard of the annual Super Bowl and the February 2004 Janet Jackson/Justin Timberlake half-time show – or I should say half-time *showing*. I'm referring to the one-second exposure, to 100 million American television viewers, of Janet's right nipple, which ended up costing the broadcaster a $500,000 fine. Almost no one commented on the lead-up sexualized song and dance that the couple did, with its suggestion of coercion and submission; but the moment a breast showed up, clearly the Republic was threatened with collapse.

126. Camerlengo M. NFC Divisional Picks. RealGM Football, January 11, 2006.

127. Silverman S. Star talks about her surgery. *PeopleNews*, March 27, 2006. Excerpt: "Phoning her [television] cohosts on *The View* Monday morning, Starn assured Meredith Vieira, Joy Behar and Elisabeth Hasselbeck [see log entries for June 7 and October 23, 2005] that 'I did not almost die. I had a boob lift. I thought it would be nice to call you guys this morning and keep you abreast of the situation.' She also admitted she'd gotten implants because she wanted her breasts to be 'perky'. Asked why she underwent the elective procedures, Jones Reynolds, 44, explained that she needed the change following her recent 150-lbs. weight loss. 'Will we be able to touch them?' Hasselbeck asked. Jones Reynolds replied, 'Elisabeth, you are such a freak.' But, she added, 'You'll be able to see them. They're just normal boobs. It's not that I went and got triple Ds.' "

128. PRWeb Press Release Newswire. Breast cancer site to remain 'under construction': by its readers, January 14, 2006.

129. http://www.breastcancerinformationsite.com/

130. Nature's Herbal Remedies Online, Allnut Enterprises http://www.naturesherbalremediesonline.com/Contact_Us.html .

131. Gupta M. Breast Cancer Information http://www.breastcancerinformationsite.com/Breast_Cancer_Information_For_Beginners.html.

132. Ksl.com News, Salt Lake City, Utah, January 15, 2006.

133. *Southern Standard*, McMinnville, Tennessee, USA, January 16, 2006.

134. New Delhi TV Ltd. China recalls dangerous infant formula, February 17, 2006.

135. Maclean's, http://www.macleans.ca/topstories/health/article.jsp?content=20060220_121862_121862, February 18, 2006.

136. Peart K. Village breastfeeding dilemma. *Herald Sun* (Melbourne), March 1, 2006.
137. Bunce J, Gallagher H. Netballer mum wins breastfeeding battle. *The Courier-Mail* (Brisbane), March 1, 2006.
138. PR Newswire. *National survey reveals need for DHA education among new moms.* Bright Beginnings Nutritionals, Gordonsville, Virginia, March 15, 2006.
139. PR Newswire. *It's Only Natural. New Moms Want Organic Infant Formula Choice for Babies.* PBM Products, LLC, Gordonsville, Virginia, March 29, 2006.
140. Ibid.
141. Lovel J. *Bright Beginnings Breaks Multimedia Campaign.* ADWEEK. COM, February 10, 2005.
142. PR Newswire, March 15, 2006, op. cit.
143. The Cochrane Collaboration http://www.cochrane.org/docs/descrip.htm is an international non-profit and independent organization, dedicated to making up-to-date, accurate information about the effects of health care available worldwide. It produces and disseminates systematic reviews of healthcare interventions and promotes the search for evidence in the form of clinical trials and other studies of interventions.
144. Simmer K. Longchain polyunsaturated fatty acid supplementation in infants born at term, op. cit.

Part three

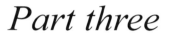

6. The Formula War

In terms of popular awareness in industrialized countries, especially those under the Anglo-Saxon arc, of the problems associated with inappropriate child feeding, the last three decades have been marked by a major clash of feeding cultures. What to say about a small group of people who set out to save mothers and children from commercial come-ons by doing battle with so-called free-market capitalist principles? These years of David vs. Goliath political activism – shoestring-budget NGOs battling large and deep-pocket commercial interests and their unfettered merchandising of industrially prepared breast-milk substitutes – have unquestionably resulted in heightened awareness of the dangers of artificial feeding in resource-poor and environmentally unsafe conditions. Indeed, had it not been for this broad-based and diverse consumer coalition, it is virtually certain that today there would be no internationally recognized standards against which the appropriate marketing and distribution of breast-milk substitutes could be gauged (even if these standards are often more honored in the breach than in the observance). Moreover, now that the standards are in place it is these same NGOs that serve as combined watchdog, goad and moral conscience for both the commercial interests and the regulatory authorities ostensibly charged with overseeing the standards' application. According to Saul Alinsky,[1] power goes to two poles: to those who've got money and to those who've got people. But even the most moral high-minded strategies can have unintended and unwanted consequences. For example increasing awareness of the problems associated with artificial feeding in conditions of relative poverty might well have little or no impact on attitudes toward breastfeeding – and thus its increased prevalence and duration – in conditions of relative wealth. This happens because, perversely, some observers arrive at the totally unwarranted conclusion that, unlike people living in poverty, the relative rich are somehow able to deviate, with impunity, from our species' pre-established nutritional and nurturing path.

Many consider that the first shot in the Formula War was fired in 1939 when doctor-to-the-poor Cecily Williams,[2] speaking at the Singapore Rotary Club, declared that "misguided propaganda on infant feeding should be punished as the most miserable form of sedition, and these deaths should be regarded as murder."[3] With formula promotion in resource-poor settings picking up in the 1960s, so, too, did criticism of artificial feeding and marketing, including Derrick Jelliffe's coining of the evocative term "commerciogenic malnutrition" in 1968 to describe what he saw as the result of unregulated marketing of infant formula among the poor;[4] a feature article in the New Internationalist in 1973 calling for a campaign to stop formula promotion; and publication by the British NGO War On Want[5] in 1974 of a report on infant malnutrition and the promotion of artificial feeding in the Third World called *The Baby Killer.* When the report was distributed later that year by the Third World Action Group in Switzerland as *Nestlé tötet Babys* [Nestlé kills babies], the Nestlé company sued for libel because of the pamphlet's title, the charge that its practices were unethical and immoral, the allegation that the company was directly responsible for the deaths of thousands of babies, and the allegation that it employed salesgirls dressed in nurses' uniforms.[6] Nestlé achieved something of a Pyrrhic victory – the defendants were found guilty of libel for the title only and fined a token sum; but the judge suggested that the company pull up its corporate socks by modifying its marketing practices. Next up: the Infant Formula Action Coalition (INFACT) launched the Nestlé Boycott in the USA in 1977 "to protest against Nestlé's unethical marketing."[7] With the exception of a four-year suspension (1984-1988) "to allow Nestlé time to put its promises into practice,"[8] the boycott has simmered ever since.

Other milestones in the Formula War include a hearing in the US Senate (May 1978) chaired by Senator Edward Kennedy that was billed as an "examination of the advertising, marketing, promotion, and use of infant formula in developing nations";[9] an international meeting on infant and young child feeding (October 1979) organized jointly by WHO and UNICEF that was attended by some 150 representatives of governments, organizations of the United Nations system and other intergovernmental bodies, nongovernmental organizations, the infant-food industry and experts in related disciplines;[10] the formation, immediately following the joint WHO/UNICEF meeting, of the International Baby Food Action Network (IBFAN)[11] by six of the NGOs present there; the World Health Assembly's endorsement (May 1980) in their entirety of the joint meeting's statement and recommendations (which had been agreed by consensus) and its request that an international code of marketing of infant formula and other products used as breast-milk substitutes be prepared in close consultation with WHO Member States and with all other parties concerned;[12] and the Health Assembly's adoption (May 1981) of the International Code of Marketing of Breast-milk Substitutes, in the form of a recommendation (with only one government voting against, the USA). On this occasion, Governments were called upon to take action to give effect to the Code "as appropriate to their social and legislative framework, including the adoption of national legislation, regulations or other suitable measures."[13]

Infant-food manufacturers do – and generally do very well – what manufacturers of consumer products of every type have always done:

- They identify markets based on existing needs.
- They seek to create new needs and fill them.
- They try to increase the size of the overall market.
- They attempt to increase their market share over that of their competitors.

There is no ambiguity about commercial encroachment on the child-feeding ideal. Indeed, commercial interests are shameless in their efforts to profit, literally and figuratively, from the way much of contemporary society is presently configured to favor use of their products at Mother Nature's expense. And commercial interests are of course only too happy to nudge society along by helping to ensure a continuation of a status quo that is so favorable – indeed compelling – to regular and repeated use of their products.

It is thus indisputable that the processed-food industry is actively engaged in creating, structuring, consolidating and expanding a market that is favorable to infant formula *for that is what commercial interests of every type do the world over*. But please, let's avoid the classic blunder of single-factor analysis by recalling that commercial interests don't operate in a vacuum. The contrast provided by two sets of relatively prosperous European countries with highly educated populations illustrates this point well.

First, let's take a look at France and Ireland which, in addition to being both modern and materially affluent, have at least one other trait in common – *miserly* ever-breastfed rates. On average, only one out of two children in France[14] and just over four out of ten (43%[15]) children in Ireland (up from 33.9% in 1993 and 39.1% in 2001[16]) ever see even a drop of breast milk (only 23% of Irish babies are still breastfeeding at six weeks postpartum[17] whereas the average duration in France is ten weeks[18]).

Next, let's have a look at Norway and Sweden, where more than 98% of newborns are routinely put to the breast within an hour of birth and 72% of babies in Sweden[19] (up from about 50% before implementation of the Baby-friendly Hospital Initiative in all maternity services[20]) and 80% in Norway[21] are still breastfeeding at six months (36% in Norway at one year).[22]

Looking at these twin polar opposites, are we then to conclude that French and Irish mothers somehow love their babies less than Norwegian and Swedish mothers do? Or perhaps that the formula reps in Paris and Dublin are more enthusiastic and consequently more effective in hawking their wares than their counterparts are in Oslo and Stockholm?

I presume that you've already supplied your own answer to the question about mothers' love. As for formula reps, my take is that they work as hard in both environments but with one vital difference. Those in Norway and Sweden face a formidable wall of society-wide *awareness* in terms of the preferred child-feeding mode. Meanwhile, their counterparts in France and Ireland continue to ride a wonderful wave of relative society-wide *ignorance* in this regard.

Some have suggested that the contrast has to do with women working outside the home. But this notion breaks down if we consider that until recently Ireland had the *lowest* rate (30% in 1994)[23] of female participation in the labor force in Western Europe even as Sweden had the *highest* (90% in 1994).[24] And until the mid-1990s Irish mothers were staying home – and still formula-feeding their babies – in significant numbers (70% from birth in 1995).[25]

Similarly, some say that it's thanks to Sweden's generous parental leave provisions that mothers breastfeed the way they do. These provisions certainly serve as a facilitator;[26] but my understanding is that they are themselves the result of a strong and coherent family policy, including protection and support of breastfeeding, that serves more as guarantor than primary motivator.

Discussions that I've had over the years with knowledgeable informants have helped me to understand that it was mainly Swedish mothers who took back breastfeeding in the 1970s. Moreover, far from leading a counterrevolution, the national health authorities and the medical community found themselves having to do some fancy footwork to catch up with one; women themselves had made their decision and it was they who took responsibility for fleshing out what most Swedes now take for granted – and the entire society and its multiple public and private institutions are structured to practice and sustain. Breast is best? Sure, why not; but in context this slogan hardly has the same mournful ring of the isolated believer's mantra in the land of an unconvinced majority, or the same hypocritical edge coming from manufacturers of "second-best" infant formula. Indeed, across Swedish society breast milk for children couldn't be any more normal *and* normalized than herring, flatbread and aquavit are for adults. That's just the way things are.

In contrast, I remember an earnest conversation I had with a number of irate members of La Leche League France in November 1993 on the occasion of this group's fifteenth anniversary. This truly courageous band of pioneers was feeling especially isolated at the time. Their efforts to gain official recognition, even a modest measure of no-cost moral support, from the national health authorities and the mainline medical community were bearing very little if any visible fruit, and their consequent discouragement was palpable. "And the pediatricians," one member practically hissed, "they're the worst!" My observation, then as now, goes like this.

In surveying the health-professional horizon, it's essential to bear in mind a basic sociocultural fact. With only the occasional exception, well before French pediatricians ever went to medical school or began to specialize in pediatrics, they were little girls and little boys growing up and coming of age in an ambient culture that was at best indifferent to – and at worst actively hostile toward – breastfeeding. And notwithstanding some notable exceptions, the medical schools and hospitals in which pediatricians trained and qualified were less change agents than compliant mirrors of the larger society in which they functioned. In fact, I would say that this unflattering picture is not only entirely consistent with the attitudes toward breastfeeding in most of contemporary France but that anything else would constitute an anomaly.[27]

Perhaps the *real* problem then with breastfeeding in France and Ireland is the fact that the French and Irish live there!

As an aside, I don't know whether to qualify it as coincidence or irony, but Ireland (1.99) and France (1.90) currently have the highest fertility rates of the European Union's 25 member countries[28] (in 2004 the rate in Australia was 1.77[29] [the same as in the UK[30]] and 2.07 in the USA). Maybe it's the result of nothing more complex than lack of lactational amenorrhea.[31]

Fortunately, all is not lost if you consider the hopeful news that the Irish Minister for Health and Children announced in Dublin Castle in June 2004 – the launching of a Blueprint for Action to protect, promote and support breastfeeding across 28 European countries.[32]

I'd like to suggest another tack to stimulate your thinking. Picture yourself participating in a child-feeding workshop, using a classic learning tool whereby small groups are formed to discuss a given topic. Here's your two-part assignment for this occasion.

First, imagine being asked to design a society-wide program, cutting across all sectors, especially education, health and social welfare, and main socioeconomic, political, ethnic and religious lines, with a single objective – *reducing by half* the ever-breastfed rates in Norway and Sweden in the space of a single generation. How would you go about doing this?

Next, imagine being asked to perform a similar exercise with a single major difference. The aim this time would be to design the same sort of society-wide program whose objective would be to *double* the ever-breastfed rates in France and Ireland, once again in the space of a single generation. How do you suppose you would go about doing that?

My point here is quite basic really; it goes back to what I said earlier about avoiding the classic blunder of single-factor analysis and recalling that commercial interests don't operate in a vacuum. Moreover, defining child-feeding options mainly in terms of Mother Nature versus the synthetic dream merchants – formula manufacturers that is – in effect lets the rest of society, including you and me, off the hook. Countering and curbing commercial interests are certainly necessary actions in context; so by all means let's remain vigilant regarding the supply side of the artificial-feeding equation. But let's also deal realistically with the demand side – the countless complex cultural determinants of child-feeding behavior.

Thus, perhaps the most important lesson we can learn from a cross-cultural perspective is that the revolution still to come in any environment with low breastfeeding rates is stillborn in the absence of a balanced look at infant-feeding practices in their everyday social context. Where infant-feeding behavior is concerned, there is too much confusion between symptoms and causes. There is also too much uncertainty about which forces in society are leading, which forces are following and which forces may be doing a bit of both. A critical eye is called for to help us see through the rhetorical fog.

Battling formula suppliers can be an exciting, even adrenaline-pumping, way to focus our energy. Unless demand gets its due, however, fighting supply is pitifully inadequate. Worse, it can be misleading and even counterproductive in terms of achieving what I believe should be our common goal – more and longer breastfeeding – and our common objective – entire societies that are geared to supporting the biological norm for the young of our species. Attempts to micromanage the activities and actions of formula producers, distributors and retailers is a dubious investment of scarce resources in the absence of a simultaneous focus on increasing awareness not just among mothers and health professionals but the entire society.

More to the point, however, a prescription for change in feeding behavior that focuses primarily on commercial interests and is filtered through a regulatory prism is also doomed to failure. Instead of more and longer breastfeeding, consistent with elementary principles of the economics of scarcity – and failing a change in values and expectations – pressure of this type results mainly in making artificial feeding still more expensive by acting like a surcharge on an airline ticket to cover rising fuel prices. Manufacturers always pass onto customers the additional cost of doing business in a more restricted marketplace (perversely, we also know that increased cost can make virtually any product still more attractive to at least some people). Ironically, already hugely inferior substitute nutrition can thus become even less adequate as a result of increasing consumer propensity to misuse a product by over-diluting it.

Infant formula's inflated market value and the still widespread prevalence of artificial feeding in many environments have resulted in unmistakable signs of increasing interest in formula as a criminal commodity (see chapter 5). The negative implications just for nutrition and food safety of this extra-legal market evolution only increase the serious health risks to which this highly vulnerable consumer subgroup is already exposed.

Putting out of business opium poppy farmers and their intermediaries in the Golden Triangle by destroying both plant and product and imprisoning Cali coca cartel kingpins is one thing; reducing demand for heroine and cocaine production and the social inequities driving their illicit importation, sale and use in London, Melbourne, New York, Paris or Toronto is quite another. If a balanced and integrated approach is required to reduce both the supply of and demand for illicit drugs, why should it be any different for infant formula?

I recognize that my analogy is imperfect. After all, infant formula, used properly within carefully defined limits, provides a positive, even life-sustaining, image – much as bottled oxygen does for someone in need of a fresh-air substitute or an insulin pump for a diabetes sufferer. On the other hand, would anyone seriously suggest that healthy people should use bottled oxygen in preference to fresh air or insulin-pump therapy in place of a normally functioning pancreas?

I repeat an earlier observation. My conclusion that artificial feeding is the result of society-wide ignorance is based on a single universal constant across time and geography – that with only the rarest of exceptions *all* mothers love their children and want what is best for them, which is always culturally determined. Thus, in the past as in the present and doubtless in the future, a woman's reason for failing *to* breastfeed as much as failing *at* breastfeeding relates, first and foremost, to her everyday sociocultural reality.

Infant-formula manufacturers know that it is consumers who are the ultimate arbiters of product and brand success. They know, too, that their approach has to be consumer-driven or, quite simply, it will not work.

Consequently, the most efficient and effective way to reduce the supply of infant formula is to reduce the demand for infant formula; and the most efficient and effective way to reduce demand for infant formula is to increase demand for breast milk.

But when I say "efficient and effective," please don't conclude that I'm implying "spontaneous and trouble-free." In the complex social environments in which we live, I recognize that often it's a very hard struggle indeed – one mother and one child at a time.

For a long time now, I've been anxious about the impact of what I refer to as a "reverse checklist," which operates most effectively at a subconscious level. I'm sure you're familiar with the original model, which goes like this.

In resource-poor settings, artificial feeding is dangerous, even deadly, because people don't have enough money to buy and use enough of a good substitute feeding product, their water is contaminated, they can't read or follow accurately product-mixing instructions, their general level of hygiene is poor, they have no refrigeration, their feeding bottles and artificial nipples (teats) are of inferior quality, and household fuel to sterilize bottles and nipples is scarce.

All things considered, this catalogue of catastrophe is accurate as far as it goes. Its main drawback is that it doesn't go far enough. The modified model – the one causing me anxiety – goes like this.

Many people living in conditions of relative wealth appear to have naively concluded that, as far as they *personally* are concerned, artificial feeding is quite adequate and safe because they have enough money to buy a good-quality substitute feeding product, their water is clean, they can easily read and accurately follow product-mixing instructions, their general level of hygiene is good, they have refrigeration, their feeding bottles and nipples are of superior quality and household fuel is plentiful. In a word, they're home free. By implication then, people in poor settings will need to breastfeed just until they have a viable alternative.

This point is convincingly made by the startlingly positive news out of Ghana that was widely – and rightly – trumpeted by the British government's Department for International Development: that breastfeeding in the first hour of life could save almost one million babies' lives each year.[33] What's my problem? Just this: The groundbreaking research, which is described as the first study to assess the effect on newborn survival rates of when mothers start to breastfeed, was conducted among nearly 11,000 breastfeeding babies in Ghana. Unfortunately, both the press release and the published journal account[34] limit discussion of the study's implications to, literally, "poor countries," whether in Africa or elsewhere. There is no mention, *not one word,* of breastfeeding's implications in "non-poor" environments, including Great Britain. While possibly of less consequence in the journal article, my fear is that, to the extent that press releases like this one are picked up by the popular media, the result is once more to implicitly confirm for general readers the uninformed stereotype of breastfeeding's being *terribly* important for babies *out there* in poor countries but without all that much significance for babies at home.

Infant-food manufacturers have eagerly exploited this bogus dichotomy, particularly since the advent of the International Code, by distinguishing for marketing purposes between their conduct in so-called developing and developed countries and promoting "informed choice" in the latter group (see observations about "informed choice" in chapter 3). At its most simplistic, the rarely explicitly stated but consistently reinforced indirect message is this: At the end of the day, while breastfeeding is admittedly good for babies in general, it is in fact crucial only for babies in poor countries. Artificial feeding in rich countries – or among elites in poor countries – presumably carries no price tag beyond the cost of an infant formula and the equipment with which to mix and feed it safely.

Commercial interests have refined to an art form the variety and subtlety of the "information" on infant feeding they provide health professionals and the general public alike. However, all manage to convey a single simple idea: Not only is it all right for you to substitute for breast milk; in fact, it doesn't really matter one way or the other provided that you buy a good product, your water is clean, you wash your hands and you follow mixing instructions.

Failing a serious challenge to the status quo in bottle-feeding cultures, no matter how egregious violations of the International Code are to us, they will not only go unpunished; more to the point, with rare exceptions they will also go virtually unnoticed, as much by the supposedly competent national authorities as by health professionals and most members of the general public. My reasons for saying this are many, but my first concerns what I believe is the International Code's leading underpinning principle – human milk's unique, species-specific properties and the inescapable implications for the health of all people throughout the life course. Regardless of how clear this underpinning principle is to you and me, widespread ignorance of it elsewhere translates into a primary barrier to more and longer breastfeeding where too many people "just don't get it" as far as respect for the biological norm for feeding the young of our species is concerned.

Experience suggests that the greater the public awareness of the significance of breast milk and breastfeeding, the more effective – and the less politically contentious – is giving effect to the International Code to deal with the supply side of the artificial-feeding equation. However, to the extent that the demand side is neglected or even ignored, we risk seeing nothing more than half-hearted attempts at Code implementation if that. And as noted above, this Code Lite approach also results more in increasing the cost of doing business in a restricted marketplace than in boosting the prevalence and duration of breastfeeding. In the absence of collective awareness that not breastfeeding very long or at all is worth bothering about, governments are acting consistently not only with prevailing political pressure and what it means to be commercial-interest friendly – which by definition all governments are – but also in ignorance of the true cost of the life-long health implications of more or less breastfeeding.

It may sound frustratingly circular, but experience also shows this: We are unlikely to see adequate measures widely adopted to protect, promote and support breastfeeding – for example broad-based community support for mothers and babies, health-professional training consistently imbued with suitable messages, baby-friendly maternity environments, maternity protection in the workplace, and appropriate marketing and distribution of breast-milk substitutes – until society and its leaders first embrace the proposition that routinely feeding a breast-milk substitute represents a significant deviation from the biological norm for the young of our species that carries with it serious consequences throughout the life course.

Politicians typically distinguish themselves as short-term thinkers and planners. Indeed, few are elected or re-elected on any other basis. Political promises, whether for less crime, safer streets or more chickens in a greater number of pots, if not exactly for today or tomorrow, then are made at least with an eye on next week, next year or next election.

The interplay of political and economic forces, including traditional capitalist free-market principles, helps explain why food manufacturers typically have the upper hand in the retail child-feeding market. There is a natural – and, heretofore at least, for the most part invisible – breastfeeding constituency of mothers and children; but food manufacturers are the only uniquely focused organized force competing in both the ideas and product marketplace for a bigger slice of Mother Nature's market share. But as in the twin polar opposites described above – France and Ireland on the one hand and Sweden and Norway on the other – factoring in levels of public awareness and predominant societal attitudes is essential to understanding how this competition is perceived and how successful it's finally going to be.

I am struck by the number of people who naively invoke the "intuitive" desire and authority of the state – read: the political will – to protect, promote and support breastfeeding in isolation from the larger socioeconomic context. (This is similar to the implicit assumption that pediatricians, as a group, should somehow be "naturally" inclined to such a bias.) The formal endorsement of countless breastfeeding-related international recommendations, declarations, resolutions and strategies notwithstanding, I draw attention once again to the fact that all governments everywhere are commercial-interest friendly. And commercial interests are able to exercise the level of influence they do with governments because of the indispensable role they play in areas crucial to the health of national economies, for example employment creation and revenue generation, and their contribution to a positive balance of payments. Left to their own devices, the artificial-feeding market forces *currently* at work in many environments thus easily manage to trump Mother Nature time and again.

As described in chapter 8, my view is that the primary reason for all this is a general lack of awareness among politicians and other decision-makers of the *true* impact of more or less breastfeeding and therefore the full economic implications for the entire society. While denial or minimization of responsibility may conceivably be understood to be in the short-term combined financial interests of governments, commercial food interests and even some health-care providers, it's clear that in the longer term these same forces are uniformly bad for society as a whole. (In the USA, which in 2006 ranked higher in infant mortality than 41 other countries or territories,[35] Palmer has conservatively estimated that formula feeding costs four additional lives per thousand births, which she calculated as double the risk of death for formula-fed compared to breastfed infants.[36] Meanwhile Chen and Rogan estimated that if all children were breastfed in the USA, 720 postneonatal deaths might be prevented or delayed each year.[37]) Until such time as politicians and other decision-makers pick up and act on this reality, the full-court press in favor of more and longer breastfeeding is simply not going to happen. As already noted in chapter 4, running breastfeeding's cost-benefit numbers successfully and understanding their significance accurately should serve as a tipping point for achieving the critical mass required to turn society's attitudes *and* behavior radically around. But until this happens, the deepest pockets have the biggest mouths.

The infant-formula industry's opposition to the original risk-based approach of the 2004 *Babies were born to be breastfed!* campaign in the USA (see chapter 7) is one of the more egregious examples of manufacturers' tactical cleverness and political influence; but it was at least predictable in context.[38] However, the virtually identical position[39] adopted by the American Academy of Pediatrics suggests at minimum a curious bit of institutional schizophrenia at the same time as the Academy's latest (and generally excellent) supportive statement on breastfeeding is being quoted the world over.[40] Meanwhile, the US Department of

Agriculture continues to provide huge quantities of free formula – at taxpayers' expense – for nutritionally at-risk infants in low-income households (more than half a billion dollars worth in 1993[41] and currently more than half of all infant formula sold in the USA[42]) even as the USDA commissions credible research on the savings that could be realized by increasing breastfeeding's prevalence and duration[43] (see chapter 8) and the impact of the workplace environment on breastfeeding duration,[44] and CDC's Office of Minority Health strives to eliminate disparities in infant mortality – more than twice the national average in some cases[45] – among the very socioeconomic groups[46] that are some of WIC's biggest infant-formula customers. This is gloomy testimony concerning a public health establishment that seems unwilling to embrace, without reservation, the notion that large-scale non-emergency artificial feeding is very risky business indeed.

It's easy for an informed pro-breastfeeding minority to become indignant at formula manufacturers and to view their behavior as morally culpable. Don't they *knowingly* do things that harm our children and mothers and aren't they *consciously* shirking their responsibility when promoting artificial feeding? Some observers are convinced that despite this awareness infant-formula manufacturers' shameless greed motivates them to seek short-term gain by enticing mothers to use their artificial feeding products in place of Mother Nature's Own.

Perhaps; but I think the question is considerably more complex than that. Moreover, in the absence of greater society-wide awareness, can companies bear all the blame for acting consistently with the rudimentary capitalist ethic and modus operandi? After all, businesses exist to make a profit for their owners.

In one direct sense, then, the buying public is as responsible for creating, accepting and maintaining an artificial child-feeding status quo as are formula manufacturers themselves. And if you think that this sounds like I'm playing a blame-the-victim game, I'll say it one more time: Commercial interests don't operate in a vacuum. It still takes two to tango.

Feeding problems and polarizing debates might well involve selfish behavior on the part of some individuals who advance their own interests while knowingly damaging the health of children and mothers. For the most part, however, such behavior cannot be so simplistically imputed to selfish manufacturers who reprehensibly profit at the expense of consumers. By the same token, it should come as no surprise to formula manufacturers that when they deviate from internationally agreed principles concerning the marketing of their products,[47] they are provoking the wrath of people whose knowledge, awareness and values lead them to adopt radically different conclusions regarding appropriate behavior in the marketplace.

Who then is living in denial? Broadly speaking, two groups I believe: first, governments that continue to ignore the implications of what they regularly pay lip-service to ("breast is best" and all that) in terms of artificial feeding's harmful consequences throughout the life course, including increased morbidity and mortality (governments are fast running out of excuses for not being better informed and acting accordingly in public-policy terms); and, second, those who focus on the marketing of breast-milk substitutes, as if in isolation, and fail to pay adequate attention to other key forces in society that significantly delay or prevent altogether a return to the biological feeding norm.

Just as governments and politicians have their roles to play, we as members of the general public bear a measure of responsibility, too. No widget maker has ever continued for very long producing widgets for which there is little or no market. Only when the public stops buying and pressures its politicians into demanding changes in the direction of what is considered responsible behavior that enhances public health – think more seat-belt and less tobacco use – will companies behave differently. Until then, don't expect them to be operating as charities in violation of their first responsibility to shareholders; or governments to be throttling a short-term cash cow in the absence of economic and political forces demonstrating awareness of what is *really* at stake in terms of the negative consequences for the entire society of routine non-emergency artificial feeding.

Consider for a moment why anyone would *knowingly* do something harmful to society as a whole or to one of its most vulnerable groups – children – or to a large proportion of over half its adult members – women. While denial or minimization of responsibility might be to the myopic short-term financial advantage of special interests (including food manufacturers, and employers and health services that have yet to grasp fully breastfeeding's significance), clearly they are bad for society as a whole. This is why education in the broadest sense of the term remains central to protecting or reverting to breastfeeding as the child-feeding norm; and why our attention must never stray from culture and society which, together, are responsible for producing and sustaining the complex value system that results in more – or variously less – breastfeeding by the mothers and children in their midst.

Should the Formula War continue? In fact, some observers have concluded that it's the right battle but the wrong war. I'll put it this way: Taking on the synthetic dream merchants implies considerably more than a regulatory frontal assault on supply; we also need to decrease demand for the synthetic dream. And this can be done only by overcoming ignorance of human milk's unique species-specific properties and the inescapable implications for the health of all people throughout the life course.

I believe it's essential that we remain big-picture strategists and that turning things around can happen only with a variety of tools, ideas and approaches employed synergistically. But whatever your view, I think you'll agree that we've finally begun to understand the monumental impudence and fundamental folly of trying to pull a fast one on Mother Nature by routinely deviating from the biological norm for feeding the young of our species. Now, for the sake of all our children, it's time we made amends and moved on.

References
1. Born in Chicago, Saul Alinsky (1909-1967) was a community organizer and social reformer who developed strategies and tactics for converting the energy of grassroots groups into effective activism.
2. For a detailed chronology of this and related events, see Baby Milk Action http://www.babymilkaction.org/pages/history.html.
3. As cited by Palmer G. in: *The Politics of Breastfeeding*, London, Pandora, 1993, p. 218.
4. Jelliffe D. Commerciogenic Malnutrition? Time for a Dialogue. *Food Technology*, February 1971, pp. 55-56.
5. War On Want http://www.waronwant.org/.
6. Nestlé, Baby Milk Issue Facts, History http://www.babymilk.nestle.com/History/.
7. Baby Milk Action, op. cit. http://www.babymilkaction.org/pages/history.html.
8. Ibid.
9. Committee on Human Resources, United States Senate. *Marketing and promotion of infant formula in the developing nations.* Washington, DC, U.S. Government Printing Office, 1978, 1498 pages.
10. World Health Organization. *International Code of Marketing of Breast-milk Substitutes.* Geneva, 1981, Introduction, p. 6.
11. With regional coordinating offices in Africa, Asia/Pacific, Europe, Latin America/Caribbean and North America, IBFAN consists of more than 150 groups worldwide http://www.ibfan.org/.
12. *International Code of Marketing of Breast-milk Substitutes*, op. cit., pp. 6-7.
13. Ibid., paragraph 11.1.
14. Haute Autorité de Santé, Association française de Pédiatrie Ambulatoire. Rapport d'élaboration de référentiel d'évaluations de pratiques professionnelles. *Allaitement maternel suivi par la pédiatrie.* Juillet 2005.
15. Ring E. Births to single mothers double over last 15 years. *The Irish Examiner*, January 24, 2006.
16. Condon D. Caesareans, home births increase. http://www.irishhealth.com/, May 3, 2005.

17. Condon D. Breastfeeding Support. http://www.irishhealth.com/, November 24, 2005.
18. Castetbon K, Dupont N, Hercberg S. Bases épidémiologiques pour la surveillance de l'allaitement maternel en France. *Revue Epidémiologique de la Santé Publique*, 2004, 52: 475-483.
19. Official Statistics of Sweden. The National Board of Health and Welfare, Centre for Epidemiology, Stockholm. *Breast-feeding, children born 2000*, page 8 http://www.sos.se/FULLTEXT/42/2002-42-7/2002-42-7.pdf.
20. Yngve Hofvander, Emeritus Professor of Pediatrics, Department of Women's and Children's Health, Uppsala University, Uppsala, Sweden (personal communication).
21. National Board of Health statistics cited by Gro Nylander in: Longer breastfeeding best, *Aftenposten* English Web Desk, November 2, 2005 http://www.aftenposten.no/english/local/article1147722.ece.
22. Ibid.
23. Clarity J. In Ireland, women's movement stalls. *International Herald Tribune*, November 4, 1994.
24. Durand C. Etre père en Suède [Being a father in Sweden]. *Femina*, April 2, 1995, pp. 14-17.
25. Consumers' Association of Ireland. Baby food. What is best to make baby grow. *Consumer Choice*, July 1994.
26. Galtry J. The impact on breastfeeding of labour market policy and practice in Ireland, Sweden, and the USA. Social Science and Medicine, 2003, 57(1):167-177.
27. Unfortunately, the situation is not much better in other settings over time as noted in the following examples. Spear HJ. Baccalaureate nursing students' breastfeeding knowledge: A descriptive survey. *Nurse Education Today*, January 2, 2006; Al-Nassaj HH, Al-Ward NJ, Al-Awqati NA. Knowledge, attitudes and sources of information on breast feeding among medical professionals in Baghdad. *Eastern Mediterranean Health Journal*, 2004, 10:871-878; Freed GL et al. National assessment of physicians' breast-feeding knowledge, attitudes, training, and experience. *Journal of the American Medical Association*, 1995, 273(6):472-476 ; Barnett E, Sienkiewicz M, Roholt S. Beliefs about breastfeeding: a statewide survey of health professionals. *Birth*, 1995, 22(1):15-20; and World Health Organization. Information and attitudes among health personnel about infant-feeding practices. *Weekly Epidemiological Record*, 1995, 17:117-120.

28. Eurostat. Statistics in focus. Population and social conditions, 15/2005. *Population in Europe 2004 – first results* http://epp.eurostat.cec. eu.int/portal/page?_pageid=0,1136184,0_45572592&_dad=portal&_ schema=PORTAL.

29. Australia's fertility rate on the rise. *The Sydney Morning Herald*, November 16, 2005.

30. National Statistics. Rise to 1.77 children per woman in 2004 http://www. statistics.gov.uk/cci/nugget.asp?id=951.

31. A postpartum woman has at least 98% protection from pregnancy for six months when she remains amenorrheic and fully, or nearly fully, breastfeeds. Bellagio Consensus, August 1988. http://www.fhi.org/ training/en/modules/LAM/s1pg14.htm

32. *Promotion of Breastfeeding in Europe: a Blueprint for Action*, http:// www.env-health.org/a/1283.

33. Department for International Development http://www.dfid.gov.uk/. Breastfeeding in the first hour of life could save almost one million babies' lives each year. Press Release, March 26, 2006.

34. Edmond KM et al. Delayed breastfeeding initiation increases risk of neonatal mortality. *Pediatrics*, 2006, 117(3):e380-e386.

35. The World Fact Book, Rank Order – Infant mortality rate http://www. cia.gov/cia/publications/factbook/rankorder/2091rank.html.

36. Palmer LF. The deadly influence of formula in America. A Natural Family Online Special Report http://www.naturalfamilyonline.com/5-bf/312-formula-report-2.htm.

37. Chen A, Rogan W. Breastfeeding and the risk of postneonatal death in the United States. *Pediatrics* 2004;113;435-439 http://pediatrics. aappublications.org/cgi/content/full/113/5/e435.

38. Petersen M. Breastfeeding ads delayed by a dispute over content. *New York Times*, December 4, 2003.

39. Democracy Now! Milk money: How corporate interests shaped government health policy for women, June 23, 2005.

40. American Academy of Pediatrics, Section on Breastfeeding. Breastfeeding and the Use of Human Milk. *Pediatrics* 2005;115:496-506.

41. United States Department of Agriculture, Food and Consumer Services, Office of Analysis and Evaluation, Washington, DC, 1995.

42. Oliveira V, Press M. *Sharing the economic burden: Who pays for WIC's infant formula?* Amber Waves, U.S. Department of Agriculture, Economic Research Services, September 2004 http://www.ers.usda. gov/AmberWaves/scripts/print.asp?page=/September04/Features/ infantformula.htm.

43. Weimer JP. *The economic benefits of breastfeeding: a review and analysis.* Food and Rural Economics Division, Economic Research Service, U.S. Department of Agriculture Food Assistance and Nutrition Report No. 13, March 2001.

44. Cooperative State Research, Education and Extension Service, Michigan Agricultural Experiment Station. *Does a lack of support at work reduce breast-feeding? Michigan Agricultural Experiment Station researchers receive $500,000 USDA grant to find out*, March 22, 2006.

45. The rate of infant deaths for African-Americans in California in 2003 was 12.3 per 1,000 births, the Center for Health Statistics reports. That compared to 5.2 deaths for Hispanics and 4.5 for whites. McCockran R. Breast-feeding is theme of community baby shower at Revival Center Ministries. *Vallejo Times Herald*, February 25, 2006.

46. Centers for Disease Control and Prevention, Office of Minority Health. *Eliminate disparities in infant mortality* http://www.cdc.gov/omh/AMH/factsheets/infant.htm.

47. *International Code of Marketing of Breast-milk Substitutes*, op. cit., and subsequent relevant policy instruments including the *Global Strategy for Infant and Young Child Feeding*. Geneva, World Health Organization, 2003.

7. Deconstructing infant formula

One of the most important tasks at hand is to take infant formula down from its totally inappropriate nutritional pedestal. I call it deconstructing in the sense that we need to shift both popular and health-professional perceptions of infant formula from the best nutritional alternative to breast milk to the least-bad nutritional alternative to breast milk.[1] We need to adjust infant formula's warm-and-fuzzy perceived public persona – Bring in the softly lit teddy bears and whispering violins! Close in on the rocking-chair-ensconced and pearl-choker-sporting bottle-feeding mother! – and return formula use to what it is at base: an emergency nutrition intervention to prevent starvation and death.

From a commercial standpoint, one of infant formula's most important perceived comparative advantages is that in most markets – for that is what we're dealing with here, marketing – it is firmly lodged in the public consciousness as No. 2 in the child-feeding hierarchy, and a very close second to breast milk at that. I compare this strategic result to what the global rental-car company Avis has accomplished since 1962 by making a lemons-into-lemonade virtue out of being second behind the reputed market leader Hertz. Meanwhile, the Avis "We try harder!" catchphrase has become one of the most successful advertising slogans of all time.

I am intentionally excluding here the evident impact in poor environments of that classic catalogue of catastrophe – inadequate resources to obtain and use an appropriately diluted infant formula, contaminated water, faulty hygiene, inability to read and follow mixing instructions, absence of refrigeration and scarcity of household fuel. We already know what this tale of woe spells in these circumstances: disease and death on a massive – and totally predictable and unnecessary – scale. Thanks in part to one of history's longest-running consumer boycotts,[2] we're well acquainted with how artificial feeding can cause serious illness and death.

I am also purposely omitting common government- and manufacturer-ordered infant-formula recalls,[3] for example a thiamine-deficient soy-based product in Israel that resulted in hospitalization for 20 babies, irreversible brain damage for a number of others, and at least three deaths;[4] a USA-wide recall of more than 41,000 24-ounce (0.71 liter) cans of Mead Johnson Nutritionals Gentlease brand due to the presence of metal particles in some cans;[5] an unsafe level of iodine in Nestlé formula that posed a risk of pathological changes to the thyroid gland[6] in China (where half of all newborns are said to be formula-fed[7] and the total infant formula market grew by nearly 50% in the first half of 2005[8]); outdated formula still on retail shelves in four out of ten stores visited in Florida[9] and in 55 of 111 randomly checked outlets in Louisiana;[10] formula "so contaminated with flies and dirt that it could only be safely sold as animal feed" shipped from Texas to Mexico;[11] seizure of 30 million liters (31.7 million quarts) of Nestlé infant formula by police in Italy due to contamination with traces of ink used in packaging[12] (followed by the decision to recall all such formula in offset-printed cartons in Italy, France, Greece, Portugal and Spain,[13] though curiously not in the United Kingdom[14]); black impurities found in a US-made formula, Similac,[15] following a consumer boycott against Enfamil, also from the USA, that was still being distributed despite a one-month suspension due to metal particles found in some cans;[16] and scandals like the three-dozen brands of bogus formula, sold cheaply to poor farmers in eastern China (see also chapter 5), that killed at least 60 babies and resulted in severe malnutrition for hundreds more in 2004[17] (in March 2006 the Ministry of Health announced that inspectors had uncovered another bogus formula on the rural market that was "hazardously low in protein, fat, vitamin A, calcium, iron and zinc").[18]

I'm leaving out as well additional dangers like intrinsic contamination of powdered infant formula with the opportunistic pathogen *Enterobacter sakazakii*[19] and microorganisms like Salmonella. These unwanted guests sometimes cause infection and illness, including severe disease in infants, particularly preterm, low-birth-weight or immunocompromised infants; and this can lead to serious developmental sequelae and death.[20] While obviously devastating to those affected, when considered in the overall context of artificial feeding they mercifully remain relatively rare occurrences. Indeed, I liken the absence of public awareness, especially in industrialized countries, of any risk from these microorganisms to what I anticipate would be the reaction of the inhabitants of my Swiss village were I to run down Main Street frantically forewarning about the dangers *for us* of the next tsunami.

But you see, what I would really like more people to know about are the life-long health and developmental implications for millions of babies the world over of the *routine* corruption of the cellular matrix, including their guts and brains; their eyes and ears; their renal, respiratory and cardiovascular systems; and the very essence of their tissues, organs and organ systems by the everyday *non-emergency* use of infant formula that's supposedly flawless in every way – nutritionally "adequate," "perfectly" clean,[21] correctly mixed[22] and lovingly fed.[23]

And what I would also really like more people to know about are the short- and longer-term implications of routine artificial feeding for the health of many millions of women, including increased risk of pregnancy,[24] postpartum hemorrhaging, iron-deficiency anemia, hip fractures and osteoporosis,[25] breast,[26] uterine[27] and ovarian[28] cancer, and quite possibly diabetes.[29]

The truly extraordinary thing is this: All this information and considerably more – including concerns about possible fertility problems later in life due to consumption of soy infant formula[30] – is already out there and readily available in the public domain, some of it for decades; and it is being confirmed and reinforced almost daily by new studies, new evidence and new understanding about this integral part of the reproductive process on which the healthy growth and development of the infants and young children of our species depend. Indeed, you could look it up. But as English philosopher John Locke observed, it is one thing to show people that they are in error. It is quite another to put them in possession of the truth.

I'm reminded here of one of sociology's elementary principles, "A situation, defined as real, is real in its consequences," and of the "hypothesis of delusion," which is applied to psychopathology in some schizophrenic patients.[31] The ordinary dictionary meaning of "delusion" is a false belief that's maintained despite compelling evidence to the contrary. Given the mass of compelling scientific and epidemiological evidence about the harm caused by routine artificial feeding, it's hardly farfetched to qualify as collective delusion the unquestioned faith that the general public and health professionals alike in many settings continue to place in infant formula.

In fact, the perceived relative risk of routine artificial feeding in industrialized countries is extremely low to non-existent despite an avalanche of contrary evidence regularly reported in the popular media. If scientific inquiry demonstrates that "Breastfeeding 'reduces SIDS risk',"[32] it's not unreasonable to conclude that artificial feeding *increases* SIDS risk. If it's true that "Breastfed babies are less likely to die,"[33] it's not unrealistic to assume that artificially fed babies are *more* likely to die. If we can believe that "Breastfeeding decreases infant mortality,"[34] it's hardly outlandish to accept that artificial feeding *increases* infant mortality. If "Breast-feeding cuts risk of myopia,"[35] shouldn't we be trumpeting the news that "Infant formula raises risk of myopia"? And doesn't "Breast milk halves gluten intolerance risk"[36] translate into "Artificial feeding doubles gluten intolerance risk"?

The backward way these headlines are currently cast accurately mirrors the majority perception. It suggests that even when reporting hopeful news, many journalists, too, can't quite come to grips with – or even identify – the cultural chasm between normal breastfeeding as the original default child-feeding mode and normal*ized* artificial feeding. They are writing, wittingly or not, in ways that continue to mask artificial feeding's serious life-long consequences for the health of children (for example higher blood pressure in adolescents[37] and increased risk of obesity in adulthood[38]) and mothers (the link between artificial feeding and increased risk of some cancers surely ranks as one of popular health knowledge's best-kept secrets[39]).

Consider what happens when the national public health authorities in the world's largest infant formula market get behind a year-long multi-media campaign with the truly inspired title *Babies were born to be breastfed.*[40] Well, several things if you bear in mind that the launching of an ad campaign with a commercial-market value of $40 million was delayed for seven months because of intense pressure not only from infant formula manufacturers[41] (which is at least understandable) but also from the American Academy of Pediatrics (which is hardly intuitive to the uninitiated). As a result, and despite convincing research pointing to the importance of focusing on risk, the campaign's approach was changed from pointing out the *risks of formula feeding* to highlighting the *benefits of breastfeeding.*[42] This certainly isn't the tack taken in most major public health campaigns over the past, say, half-century to promote awareness about reducing health risks through public service advertisements, for example on , not smoking, and preventing underage drinking, drunk-driving and obesity.[43] Why have we made an exception for breastfeeding?

We continue to devote considerable time and other resources to singing the praises of breast milk and breastfeeding. Isn't it time we also focused on illustrating why normalized artificial feeding is next to the nadir of nutritional mediocrity and what the true – that is complete and permanent – costs are, both to individuals across the entire life course[44] and thus to society as a whole? Completion of the counterrevolution already under way will be deferred for as long as there is lack of a critical mass – an adequate proportion of the general public, health professionals and politicians that has finally grasped what routine infant formula feeding is really all about and what its true implications are in both the short and longer term.

Frequent media reports about pollutants in human milk attest to nothing more than the fact that breast milk is a convenient non-invasive means of detecting environmental pollutant load for populations as a whole.[45] The implications for feeding children are frequently secondary or ignored altogether even as reports in the popular media serve to stir passions, generate anxiety and contribute to a spike in infant-formula use.

A major article like "Toxic breast milk?"[46] appearing in a prestigious general news medium like the Sunday *New York Times Magazine* is a good example of this kind of report. From a journalistic and, I assume, scientific standpoint, it seems to be an excellent piece in every way. However, notwithstanding the author's generally enthusiastic endorsement of breastfeeding, my problem with articles like this one (and there are many) is that they rarely, if ever, help readers understand what is really going on and what in fact is being compared. Moreover, as Jack Newman not so rhetorically asks, why would everything else on Earth be polluted, even in the far reaches of the Arctic,[47] but not infant formula?[48]

Indeed, according to a recent US Senate committee report,[49] contamination with perchlorate, which is the explosive ingredient in solid rocket fuel, has been found in 34 states. Perchlorate is a thyroid toxin, and animal tests show that even small amounts can disrupt normal growth and development in fetuses, infants and children; according to the Environmental Working Group, it has been found in milk, produce and many other foods and animal feed crops from coast to coast. Meanwhile, the White House Office of Science & Technology Policy is reported to be pressuring CDC to delay the release of the study prepared at the Committee's request, which is said to describe levels that "leave no margin of safety" compared to the current risk limit.[50]

Jack Newman also makes these essential points. Toxins raise concern that the baby's cognitive ability will be affected – yet breastfed babies do better in almost every study ever published and the longer they are breastfed the better they do; and in the few that don't show better results for breastfed babies, they do at least as well. Toxins raise concern that they may affect the baby's immune system – yet breastfed babies have a better immune system and a more mature one. Toxins raise concern that they increase the risk of cancer in the baby – yet breastfed babies have a lower risk.[51]

So, not only are uninformed readers inclined to conclude that if there is *any possible danger whatsoever* of environmental pollutants in breast milk, thank goodness that "safe" infant formula will always be there to carry the day without sacrificing much at all in terms of children's health and development. In fact, based on formula's firmly fixed "good enough" position in the collective consumer consciousness, the message is much more subtle, effective and insidious than that. Many still do not appreciate that a nutritional silk purse, even a somewhat tattered one due to low concentrations of pollutants, still trumps an emergency-nutrition-intervention sow's ear every time.

When it comes to feeding babies, in purely theoretical terms there are three possibilities: breastfeeding, other feeding and no feeding. Assuming we can eliminate the last "option" on ethical grounds, it's reasonable to conclude that a baby who is denied access to breast milk, for whatever reason, is a baby who has to be fed on a breast-milk substitute. We don't need to conduct an investigation before taking action to decide *why* this is so, only observe *that* it's so and get on with feeding the best – make that the least-bad – breast-milk substitute available. The First Principles' first principle remains as intuitive as it is imperative: Feed the baby.[52]

Infant formula will sustain life in a pinch, and thank goodness this is so. But from a nutritional and developmental standpoint, not everyone has understood just how hugely inferior it is to breast milk, with negative implications for both children and their mothers – and thus the whole population – across the entire life course. The idealized view of normalized infant-formula feeding that manufacturers are so adept at portraying – and, regrettably, so many consumers, health professionals and politicians are inclined to accept – doesn't allow for even a hint of this disenchanting reality. Finally, routine non-emergency formula feeding ends up being perceived across society and culture as a perfectly legitimate, albeit second-best, source of nourishment for children instead of the vastly inferior ersatz pretender that it is.

If we wish to move infant formula, once and for all, from the kitchen pantry and permanently relegate it to where it got its start – in the medicine cabinet, *for emergency use only* – there needs to be a major shift in popular, health-professional and political thinking. In the first decade of the third millennium, deconstructing infant formula may well be our single most important priority in this connection, starting in well-to-do environments in any part of the world. It most assuredly is a pre-condition to moving to breastfeeding's next plateau – improved awareness followed by the significant behavioral change throughout society that will lead to greater prevalence and duration. We have no time to waste in achieving this goal.

References
1. The best alternative to breast milk directly from the breast of a child's own mother is, of course, breast milk provided otherwise, for example expressed breast milk, followed by milk from a human-milk bank or a healthy wet-nurse. Notwithstanding manufacturers' insistence, infant formula is thus not second but fourth in this nutritional hierarchy.

2. Nestlé Boycott. Wikipedia http://en.wikipedia.org/wiki/Nestle_boycott.

3. According to Breastfeeding.com, between 1982 and 1994 alone there were 22 significant recalls of infant formula in the USA due to health and safety problems. Seven of these recalls were classified by the U.S. Food and Drug Administration (FDA) as Class I, or potentially life threatening. The FDA Enforcement Report Index http://www.fda.gov/opacom/Enforce.html lists many more.

4. Outbreak of life-threatening thiamine deficiency in infants in Israel caused by a defective soy-based formula. *Pediatrics*, 115(2), February 2, 2005, pp. e233-e238.

5. Liu D. Metal in infant formula prompts nationwide recall. foodconsumer. org, February 24, 2006.

6. *People's Daily Online*, June 23, 2005. Beijing orders Nestle to recall questionable milk powder.

7. *People's Daily Online*, May 30, 2005. Half of China's newborns fed with infant formula powder.

8. Qingdao, China and Rockville, Maryland. Synutra International, Inc. announces new product launches. Press release, March 22, 2006.

9. WTSP TV, Tampa/St. Petersburg, 10 News Extra: Expired infant formula on store shelves, November 18, 2005.

10. Louisiana Ag inspectors find outdated baby food in 55 stores. Janet McConnaughey, Associated Press, June 30, 2005.

11. Company agrees to stop selling contaminated infant formula. El Paso, MySanAntonio.com., September 15, 2005.

12. Italian police seize contaminated Nestle baby milk, Reuters, November 22, 2005.

13. Swiss Info / Swiss Radio International. Nestlé forced to withdraw baby milk, November 23, 2005.

14. Poulter S. Contaminated baby milk stays on sale. *Daily Mail*, November 26, 2005.

15. Yon-se K. Foreign material found in another US baby formula. *The Korea Times*, March 8, 2006.

16. Yon-se K. Enfamil baby food sold despite ban. *The Korea Times*, March 9, 2006.

17. The Associated Press, 20 April 2004. Fake formula kills Chinese infants. MSNBC News http://www.msnbc.msn.com/id/4785942/.

18. Inferior infant formula reappears on market. China View, February 16, 2006.

19. Drudy D et al. *Enterobacter sakazakii*: An emerging pathogen in powdered infant formula. *Clinical Infectious Diseases*, 2006;42:996-1002.

20. FAO/WHO Expert Meeting on *E. sakazakii* and other Microorganisms in Powered Infant Formula: Meeting Report. Microbiological Risk Assessment Series No. 6, 2004, p. 37.

21. Walker M. Known contaminants found in infant formula. *Mothering*, May-June 2000 http://www.findarticles.com/p/articles/mi_m0838/is_2000_May-June/ai_62141685.

22. Fein SB, Falci CD. Infant formula preparation, handling, and related practices in the United States. *Journal of the American Dietetic Association*, 1999, 99(10):1234-1240 ("Failure to comply with recommendations was high for several practices with clear health implications").

23. Linda Folden Palmer. The deadly influence of formula in America. A Natural Family Online Special Report, December 2003 http://www.naturalfamilyonline.com/BF/200312-formula-report.htm.

24. A postpartum woman has at least 98% protection from pregnancy for six months when she remains amenorrheic and fully, or nearly fully, breastfeeds. Bellagio Consensus, August 1988. http://www.fhi.org/training/en/modules/LAM/s1pg14.htm

25. Turck D. Breastfeeding: health benefits for child and mother [Article in French]. *Archives of Pediatrics*, 2005, 12S3:S145-S165.

26. Collaborative Group on Hormonal Factors in Breastfeeding. Breast cancer and breastfeeding: collaborative reanalysis of individual data from 47 epidemiological studies in 30 countries, including 50302 women with breast cancer and 96973 women without the disease. Op. cit.

27. Okamura C et al. Lactation and risk of endometrial cancer in Japan: a case-control study. *The Tohoku Journal of Experimental Medicine*, 2006, 208(2):109-115.

28. Riman T, Nilsson S, Persson I. Review of epidemiological evidence for reproductive and hormonal factors in relation to the risk of epithelial ovarian malignancies. *Acta Obstetricia et Gynecologica Scandinavica*, 2004, 83(9):783-95.

29. Stuebe AM et al. Duration of lactation and incidence of type 2 diabetes. *Journal of the American Medical Association*, 2005; 294:2601-2610.

30. Center for the Evaluation of Risks to Human Reproduction. NTP-CERHR Expert Panel Report on the reproductive and developmental toxicity of soy formula (draft). Research Triangle Park, January 2006 http://www.thewbalchannel.com/download/2006/0316/8065400.pdf.

31. Davies M, Coltheart M, Langdon, R, Breen N. Monothematic delusions: Towards a two-factor account. In: Hoerl C, ed. *On understanding and explaining schizophrenia*, a special issue of *Philosophy, Psychiatry and Psychology*, 2001, 8(2-3).

32. *The Australian*, 29 April 2004.

33. *Washington Post*, 3 May 2004, reporting on Chen A, Rogan WJ. Breastfeeding and the risk of postneonatal death in the United States. *Pediatrics*, 2004, 113(5):e453-9.

34. Press release, National Institute of Environmental Health Science, Research Triangle Park, North Carolina, May 2, 2004, reporting on Chen A, Rogan WJ, *ibid.*

35 Breast-feeding cuts risk of myopia. *Atlanta Journal Constitution*, June 21, 2005, reporting on Chong YS et al. Association between breastfeeding and likelihood of myopia in children. *Journal of the American Medical Association*, 2005; 293:2999-3000.

36. United Press International. Breast milk halves gluten intolerance risk. London, November 15, 2005.

37. Infant feeding and components of the metabolic syndrome: findings from the European Youth Heart Study. *Archives of Disease in Childhood*, 2005; 90: 582-8.

38. Yadav M, Akobeng AK, Thomas AG. Breast-feeding and childhood obesity. *Journal of Pediatric Gastroenterology & Nutrition*. 30(3):345, March 2000.

39. Since the collaborative reanalysis of individual data on breast cancer and breastfeeding (op. cit., *Lancet*, 2002, 360(9328)203-10), I have been a guest speaker to five USA-based travelling student groups and one Swiss class, or about 130 people in all. Students were 18 to 26 years of age, more than 90% female, and many were preparing for careers in health. I used these occasions to ask the following question: Can anyone tell me about a link between breastfeeding and breast cancer? With the exception of one student, who said she thought that women who breastfed were at *increased* risk of breast cancer, no one had the slightest notion in this regard. I then used this jaw-dropping (theirs not mine) teaching moment to do two things: provide a summary of the facts of the matter and suggest it was worth pondering how a group that was so well-educated, informed, health-conscious and overwhelmingly female had arrived at adulthood totally ignorant of this vital aspect of reproductive health.

40. National Breastfeeding Awareness Campaign – Babies were born to be breastfed. A project of the U.S. Department of Health and Human Services, Office on Women's Health, 2005, http://www.4woman.gov/breastfeeding/index.cfm?page=Campaign.

41. Petersen M. Breastfeeding ads delayed by a dispute over content. *New York Times*, December 4, 2003.

42. Milk Money: How corporate interests shaped government health policy for women. Democracy Now! June 23, 2005, http://www.democracynow.org/article.pl?sid=05/06/23/1358237.

43. The Advertising Council, Inc., New York, NY http://www.adcouncil.org/campaigns/.

44. Walker M. A fresh look at the risks of artificial feeding. Child Institute, Foundation for Children http://www.childthai.org/ciec/c011.htm.

45. As one writer points out, breast-milk monitoring is not without controversy. Some women's groups suggest that informing mothers that they are passing polybrominated flame retardants, dioxin and even DDT to their babies might discourage breastfeeding. Commonweal's Sharyl Patton (http://www.commonweal.org/programs/brc/), who has worked extensively on the issue, insists that human milk is still the best choice for a baby. The information is obviously alarming, but she argues it is always better to know. Lactation proponents may object to the second point, Ms. Patton observes, but they share the same goal – we want to protect babies – and agree the answer is to stop pollution, not nursing mothers. Allen S. You are what you eat … breathe … scrub … lather … spray. The Ottawa Citizen, March 5, 2006 http://www.canada.com/windsorstar/story.html?id=1a0ccc38-194a-4f28-8e96-3e62a625b13e.

46. Florence Williams. Toxic breast milk? *New York Times Magazine*, January 9, 2005 http://www.mindfully.org/Health/2005/Toxic-Breast-Milk9jan05.htm.

47. Cone M. Polar bears face new toxic threat: flame retardants. *The Los Angeles Times*, January 9, 2006.

48. The Birth Den http://www.thebirthden.com/Newman.html, Newman J. Toxins and Infant Feeding, Handout #28, January 2005.

49. United States Senate, Committee on Appropriations. Bill S.2810 making appropriations for, among other, the Department of Health and Human Services, September 15, 2004. "The Committee is concerned about contamination due to perchlorate, which is primarily used as an oxidizer for rocket fuel and munitions. Perchlorate contamination has been discovered in 34 States and is known to have adverse health effect on pregnant women, newborns, and young children. The Committee strongly urges the CDC to conduct surveys on the level of perchlorate in humans, to provide information for assessments on a national level, and to address regional concerns in areas most affected."

50. Environmental Working Group. White House delays release of study showing toxic rocket fuel in most Americans, March 3, 2006 http://www.ewg.org/issues/perchlorate/20060303/index.php.

51. Ibid.

52. I attribute both this compelling notion and its stark formulation to self-described granny zealot and coach, Linda Smith, who is a lactation consultant in private practice in Dayton, Ohio.

8. The really big money

There are some truly outrageous claims regularly made about the value of breast milk or, more accurately, the absence of value. One of the most infuriating that I see repeatedly is that breast milk is somehow free. Ironically, breastfeeding advocates sometimes unwittingly get caught up in this foolishness, even to the point of adopting that especially ugly advertising tautology "free gift" – as opposed to the kind we pay for? While we occasionally speak about the money breastfeeding saves, we mostly ignore what breastfeeding costs. Breast milk is most assuredly not free. In fact, I would start by describing it as priceless, even as breastfeeding itself has at least three price tags directly attached: a mother's time (which far too many people erroneously consider to be on the house), the energy cost of producing milk (up to 500 kcal a day that need to come from somewhere) and the opportunity cost. You'll have no difficulty recognizing the first two tags, which are an altogether spectacular bargain when you consider the payback in terms of positive lifelong consequences for children, mothers and thus the entire society. But the third one may not be so familiar. I'm borrowing from economic theory where "opportunity cost" refers to the cost of something in terms of an opportunity forgone – for example mothers who must choose between staying at home with their children and returning to paid employment outside the home to meet their families' financial needs. As we all know from personal experience, there really is no such thing as a free lunch.

Societies that are structured in lock-step fashion to favor normalized artificial feeding will remain largely unchallenged and unchanged as long as the true economic impact of more or less breastfeeding fails to register on national radar screens. There's not much point in playing on politicians' heartstrings in attempting to gather support for breastfeeding. My view is that we need to hit them in the pocketbook instead.

Since at least the 1970s there have been numerous attempts to assess the economic value of breast milk and breastfeeding, and various aspects of the financial burden from not breastfeeding. These range from the relatively unsophisticated, including literal formula-can-counting exercises; to estimates of the total volume and value of breast milk produced in a given setting and efforts to incorporate these figures in national food accounts; to complex cost/benefit calculations based on detailed morbidity and mortality data. Here are some of the most frequently cited examples (all figures are in US$).

- In 1979 Almroth, Greiner and Latham attempted to estimate the economic value of breastfeeding in Côte d'Ivoire and Ghana. Calculated on the basis of a two-year period, the cost of artificial feeding amounted to $310 to which another $210 should be added for the cost of the time spent in breastfeeding. The sum would be almost three times higher than that for breastfeeding in the same countries.[1]

- In 1993, Bailey and Deck calculated that ear infections in the USA cost more than $1 billion annually in visits to physicians. Breastfed children have a 60% decrease in risk for ear infections compared with formula-fed infants.[2]

- In 1994, Oshaug and Botten estimated the value of milk traded in milk banks in Norway (population then 4.3 million) to have a market value of around $2.2 billion.[3] (Overall human-milk production in Norway in 2004 alone – with a population just under 4.6 million – was estimated to be 10.3 million liters [nearly 108 million quarts].[4])

- In 1994, the UK Baby-friendly Initiative reported that each 1% increase in the number of babies breastfed to three months would save the National Health Service nearly $1 million a year.[5]

- In 1995, one of the largest health care providers in the USA disclosed that infants who were breastfed for a minimum of six months generated $1,435 less in health care claims in the first year of life alone than their formula-fed counterparts.[6]

- In 1997, Riordan reported a total of $1.3 billion potential savings in health care costs in the USA using just four medical diagnoses – diarrhea, respiratory infection, diabetes mellitus, and middle-ear infection.[7]
- In 1997, Drane estimated that a minimum of $8.5 million could be saved each year in Australia (population then just under 18 million) if the prevalence of exclusive breastfeeding at three months increased from 60% to 80%.[8]
- In 1999, Ball and Wright cited additional health care costs in Arizona of between $331 and $475 over the first year of life for each never-breastfed infant.[9]
- In 2001, Weimer estimated that a minimum of $3.6 billion would be saved annually if breastfeeding were increased from the then-current US levels (64% in hospital, 29% at six months) to those recommended by the Surgeon General (75% and 50%, respectively).[10] (Meanwhile, WIC provides free formula to almost two million nutritionally at-risk infants in low-income households, or over half of all infant formula sold in the USA;[11] and the US Government Accountability Office reports that breastfeeding is less common among mothers who get federal help from WIC and that some strategies to market formula may be discouraging breastfeeding.[12])
- In 2005, Smith reported that Australian mothers produce annually 34 million liters of breast milk (about 36 million quarts). On this basis, the net economic value of breastfeeding in Australia – population today 20 million – is $1.55 billion a year.[13]

These are indeed impressive figures, even if it is not you and I who need to be convinced that acting responsibly, consistent with who and what we are as a species, could produce any other outcome. Unfortunately, this information has yet to capture adequately the attention of national and international policy-makers concerned with cost-effective decision-making. We need to ask ourselves why; but as we ponder prospects for change let's be sure not to confuse ignorance and bad management with destiny.

Perhaps the message hasn't penetrated sufficiently because it's not been adequately packaged, including by pointing out the full cost of artificial feeding, throughout the life course, for the entire society and not just the savings generated through breastfeeding. Or maybe the most compelling information has still to be assembled, analyzed, assessed and announced in convincing ways.

Just how much longer are we going to have to wait for this to happen? Not long, I believe, *provided* that recent advances in our collective science-based understanding of the health – and therefore the economic – implications of more or less breastfeeding are honestly and thoroughly assessed, convincingly presented, and taken fully into account. (In the context I'm reminded of the oft-cited aphorism attributed to former Harvard University president Derek Bok: If you think education is expensive, try ignorance.)

I'm of course referring to the continuing avalanche of truly stunning information about artificial feeding's permanent impact in terms of, for example, impaired postpartum brain development and visual acuity; increased risk of premature child mortality; increased risk for children of multiple diseases including allergies, celiac disease, diabetes, diarrheal disease, ear infection, leukemia, necrotizing enterocolitis, obesity, respiratory ailments, sepsis and urinary tract disease; increased risk in later life of cardiovascular disease; and, for mothers, increased risk of anemia and hemorrhaging, breast, ovarian and endometrial cancer, osteoporosis and rheumatoid arthritis. When these facts and figures, thoroughly evaluated and correctly correlated, finally hit the newsstands, earlier calculations are going to seem trifling indeed.

As an illustration, join me in focusing on the really big money for society as a whole in a futuristic dream sequence involving the Nobel Foundation. It's 2016 and the annual round of Nobel

Prize laureates is being announced. Since Marie Curie became the first female laureate in 1903, more than 30 women have been honored in every category but one – economics, which was first awarded in 1969. Thus, history is being made today with not one but three women, who have worked closely as a team for the last decade, achieving this distinction for the first time: Professor Guadalupe Sanchez Flores, a Mexican health economist, Phyllis Brown PhD, an American medical anthropologist, and Dr. N'sheemaehn Nanogak,[14] a Canadian First Nation nutritional epidemiologist.

The Nobel Foundation's announcement on this occasion reads as follows:

The 2016 Nobel Prize in Economics is being presented jointly to Guadalupe Sanchez Flores, Phyllis Brown and N'sheemaehn Nanogak:

- *for their pioneering empirically founded contribution to our collective understanding of the multiple, complex and lifelong economic implications of observing or disregarding the hominid blueprint for nourishing the young of our species;*
- *for their unifying theory, integrating the short- and longer-term economic implications of the impact of more or less breastfeeding on the health and cognitive development of babies, on the health of children and adults, and on the health of mothers, families and thus entire societies;*
- *for their penetrating analysis of the interdependence of early feeding patterns, and health maintenance and health expenditure throughout the life course for entire populations.*

With Dr. Nanogak providing the science base gleaned from multiple randomized trials and observational studies in high-, medium- and low-income countries; Dr. Brown drawing on a wide range of social, cultural, biological and linguistic theories and methods to better understand the factors which influence health and well-being and prevent sickness; and Professor Sanchez Flores running the numbers to tease out breastfeeding's true and complete lifelong cost/benefit implications, their groundbreaking interdisciplinary collaboration has also succeeded in integrating insights from psychological research into economic science. This concerns education in the broadest sense of the term, human judgment, and decision-making about child feeding in the presence or absence of supportive environments; risk and protective dimensions of human behavior, cultural norms and social institutions; and the opportunity costs a mother faces when forced to choose between breastfeeding her child and her role as family breadwinner.

In addition to being mothers themselves, Professor Sanchez Flores, Dr. Brown and Dr. Nanogak have for many years promoted breastfeeding in and through mother-support groups. Professor Sanchez Flores and Dr. Brown, who are long-time accredited La Leche League leaders, and Dr. Nanogak, who is an International Board Certified Lactation Consultant, regularly serve the mothers and children of their respective communities.

Who profits from breastfeeding? Not infant formula manufacturers obviously, or anyone else in the production, marketing and related services chain, including pharmaceutical companies (which of course also produce a lot of formula). And if you're sufficiently cynical, you might think that even some pediatricians and some children's hospitals don't either, at least not in the short term.

Reflect for a moment on just how much business, and what kind, would be lost – throughout society and the entire life course – if most of the world's children really *were* breastfed as recommended – exclusively for the first six months of life and thereafter, together with nutritionally adequate and safe complementary foods, for up to two years of age or beyond.[15]

Unfortunately, the true cumulative costs of artificial feeding and the savings that accrue from a greater prevalence and duration of breastfeeding remain hidden from the majority of observers. Meanwhile, many persist in the delusion that breast milk is somehow free and that large-scale normalized artificial feeding is without significant economic consequences.

Do I genuinely believe in the substance of the dream sequence I have imagined here? Leaving specifics aside for the moment – but only for a moment – as a matter of fact I do. Perhaps you've heard that popular slogan: A mind is a terrible thing to waste.[16] Let me ask you this then: What would you say are the implications of more or less breastfeeding for the world's 136 million or so new minds *every single year*?[17]

References
1. Almroth S, Greiner T, Latham M. Economic importance of breastfeeding. *Food and Nutrition* 1979; 5(2):4-10.
2. Bailey D, Deck L. *The potential health care cost of not breastfeeding.* Best Start-Kentucky, Lexington-Fayette County Health Department, 1993.
3. Oshaug A, Botten G. Human milk in food supply statistics. *Food Policy* 1994; 19(5)479-482.
4. Directorate for Health and Social Affairs, Department of Nutrition. *Utviklingen I Norsk Kosthold.* Matforsyningsstatistikk og Forbruksundersøkelser, Sosial- og helsedirektoratet, 2004, IS-1218.
5. Cited by: Breastfeeding Committee for Canada. *Cost Savings from Breastfeeding.* An annotated bibliography 1999 http://www.breastfeedingcanada.ca/html/webdoc24.html.
6. Kaiser Permanente: internal research to determine benefits of sponsoring an official lactation program http://www.visi.com/%7Eartmama/kaiser.htm.
7. Riordan J. The cost of not breastfeeding : A commentary. *Journal of Human Lactation* 1997; 13(2)93-97.
8. Drane D. Breastfeeding and formula feeding : preliminary economic analysis. *Breastfeeding Review* 1997; 5:7-15.
9. Ball TM, Wright AL. Health care costs of formula-feeding in the first year of life. *Pediatrics* 1999; (103)(4 Pt 2):870-876.

10. Weimer JP. *The economic benefits of breastfeeding: a review and analysis.* Food and Rural Economics Division, Economic Research Service, U.S. Department of Agriculture Food Assistance and Nutrition Report No. 13, March 2001.

11. Oliveira V, Press M. *Sharing the economic burden: Who pays for WIC's infant formula?* Amber Waves, U.S. Department of Agriculture, Economic Research Services, September 2004 http://www.ers.usda. gov/AmberWaves/scripts/print.asp?page=/September04/Features/ infantformula.htm.

12. United States Government Accountability Office. Breastfeeding: *Some strategies used to market infant formula may discourage breastfeeding; state contracts should better protect against misuse of WIC name.* GAO-06-282, February 2006.

13. Smith JP, Ingham LH. Mothers' milk and measures of economic output. *Feminist Economics* 2005; 11(1), March 2005, 41-46.

14. As befits a dream sequence, all three patronyms are objectively fictional. Nevertheless, anyone familiar with Mexican and American culture will easily identify with the first and second, while the last is a First Nation Canadian composite. The chickadee, called N'sheemaehn for its distinctive cries by the Anishinaubae peoples (Ojibway, Ottawa, Pottawatomi and Algonquin), is a symbol of the duty, care and responsibility that parents, guardians and the community are expected to exercise toward their children. N'sheemaehn also serves to remind humankind that accidents occur during the briefest moments of inattention; and that one will always be reminded of one's guilt should one's neglect cause harm to a child (see: http://www. utsc.utoronto.ca/~childcare/name.html). Nanogak is my way of paying tribute to Inuit storyteller and illustrator Agnes Nanogak (1925-2002).

15.   Global Strategy for Infant and Young Child Feeding, op. cit., paragraph 10.

16. "A mind is a terrible thing to waste" is the slogan of the United Negro College Fund, Fairfax, Virginia, USA http://www.uncf.org/.

17. World Health Organization, *World Health Report 2005*, Chapter 4, Attending to 136 million births, every year. Geneva, 2005.

Part four

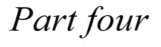

9. Metaphorically yours

I like using the ordinary to approach what is commonplace for some but still unfamiliar for others. The purpose is twofold: to show how everyday analogies, images, metaphors, similes and symbols can be used to see breast milk and breastfeeding from a fresh perspective; and to suggest how this approach in turn can help others see breast milk and breastfeeding in ways they would surely never have imagined. I include an occasional wink at the marketplace by using some cherished commercial jargon to describe what Mother Nature is up against, every day, on a very uneven playing field.

Of pleasure and pain

When I was at most 8 or 9 years old I distinctly recall seeing a woman moving down the street with pronounced difficulty. In retrospect, the word waddle comes to mind; certainly walk would have been an exaggeration. You see, the woman was decked out in the popular attire of the early 1950s that has come and gone in several sartorial swings since. She was wearing that killer combination of a very tight-fitting kick-pleat skirt and super-high spike-heel shoes – the kind that simultaneously tightens the hamstrings; thrusts outward, and conspicuously raises, the buttocks; and bends the waist unnaturally forward. And I remember making two distinct, if interrelated, observations about what I was seeing. The first was fairly explicit: Gee, she looks like she's really uncomfortable, even in pain. The second was more implicit but no less obvious: I don't understand this picture at all, but I'm sure that one day, when I'm grown up, I will. Where my first observation is concerned, countless podiatrists, rheumatologists, chiropractors and women themselves have long since confirmed my juvenile intuition. As to the second, I'm still awaiting enlightenment.

The perception of pleasure and pain – and sometimes the pleasure *of* pain – surely ranks high on the short list of ultimate human subjectivities. Pain specifically, whether its anticipation, experience or recollection, is mediated by a number of key variables; these include the sociocultural (group-imposed values and expectations), the chemical (endorphins, medication) and the experiential (learned behavior). And speaking of short lists, "sore nipples" certainly sits up there with "insufficient milk" as among the most common reasons primarily Western women give for ceasing to breastfeed. However, if all the breastfeeding women I know are to be believed, breastfeeding and pain are *not* synonymous (from an evolutionary standpoint, how could they be?). Since pre-history nipple soreness is just one more thing that more experienced mothers typically assist less experienced mothers in preventing or correcting. But I can't help but wonder how many women base their decision not to breastfeed at all on their fear of pain. So, maybe I understand a little better now what getting all gussied up in a tight skirt and high-heels means to someone who's primarily motivated by being dressed to kill at any cost – welcome to the School of Silent Sartorial Suffering – and how important it is for a breastfeeding mother to receive elementary guidance on preventing sore nipples or worse.

Cultural cover-up

What I had learned in essentially theoretical terms as a sociology undergraduate in the mid-1960s I have lived since in very dissimilar sociocultural environments: initially in the USA (where I had spent the first two decades of my life) and then in Turkey, Cameroon, Haiti and, most recently, Switzerland. Something considered "natural" and "obvious" in one cultural environment could – indeed most often is – viewed quite differently in another. This truism was effectively illustrated in a letter to *The Lancet* I saw in the early 1990s from a British obstetrician who described an experience he'd had while working in Saudi Arabia. He was making rounds one evening in the maternity wing of the ultra-modern King Faisal Specialist Hospital and Research Center in Riyadh. As he turned the corner at the bottom of a long empty corridor, he unexpectedly came, literally, face to face with a clutch of Saudi mothers visiting with each other in the hallway while breastfeeding their newborn babies. Under the circumstances, it's not difficult to imagine the scene as this lone Western male teetered awkwardly mid-stride and five startled Saudi mothers moved urgently to cover up their... faces. As to the babies, according to the obstetrician they never missed a gulp.

Flying civilly

I took my first commercial flight in 1965. In the hundreds of times I've flown since, in addition to the vastly increased number of travelers, I've seen some important changes in the size and technical enhancement of aircraft. However, thanks to uniform International Civil Aviation Organization rules applied by the world's governments, at least one aspect of air travel has remained fairly constant – the timing and content of the security briefing flight attendants provide passengers before each and every take-off.

Doubtless you already know the drill. In addition to being requested to fasten your seat belt and not to smoke, you are routinely advised that in case of a loss of oxygen in the cabin, oxygen masks will spill out automatically from an overhead compartment; and should the aircraft be forced down over water a life jacket is located under your seat.

All very reassuring information, or is it? More is probably less, especially for frequent flyers; it's unlikely that our attention is exactly riveted to messages that are repeated, if not necessarily heard, over and over again – like "breast is best" for example. In any case, I'd like to suggest a different perspective to this security briefing.

I'm reasonably certain that there are at least two key implicit assumptions in this connection that every passenger, if pressed, would readily accept. The first is that the equipment – the mask and the vest as much as the automatic oxygen delivery system – reflects the most up-to-date technology, that it is of the highest quality manufacture, that it is checked regularly by maintenance staff and replaced as needed, and that it will, indeed, work in case of emergency.

My second assumption? That we'll never actually have to use the stuff!

This is in fact an excellent way to regard infant formula. Unquestionably, for the sake of babies who have to be fed on a breast-milk substitute, we need to continue doing everything we can to ensure that formula is the *least inadequate* that nutritional science can possibly make it. And then we need to ensure that it's used *only* in an emergency.

Break glass only in case of emergency

When I worked in an office environment, there were regular fire drills to prepare us for the day that naturally we all hoped would never arrive. At one point I was also asked to serve as floor warden, and this meant that I was responsible for making sure that everyone had left the building – using the stairway of course – during what, fortunately, was never anything more serious than periodic testing of the emergency fire-alarm and evacuation systems. There were several stairways in the building; however, the one at the extreme east end, while permitting movement between floors, led only to a locked door on the ground floor. The good news was that just to the left of this locked door was a small bright-red metal box. The cover was made of glass so it was easy to see that behind it hung a key, which was readily accessible thanks to a little steel hammer mounted to one side – for use only in case of emergency of course. Infant formula also belongs behind glass, for use only in case of emergency by babies who have to be fed on a breast-milk substitute.

The sky's the limit

Think for a moment of breast milk as if it were the tallest, most aesthetically pleasing and architecturally most accomplished building the world has ever known. No one, least of all infant formula manufacturers, would dispute this grandiose image of superiority. On the contrary, formula manufacturers have a stake in perpetuating the public perception that breast milk is unquestionably the best for babies – and that formula is right behind it.

Now, even as you mouth the mantra "breast is best," think of infant formula the way manufacturers continually invite you to do – as another building which, while not quite so imposing as Mother Nature's Own, is nevertheless relatively tall, rather aesthetically pleasing, and reasonably architecturally accomplished.

No, it's not.

In fact, there's only one building on the baby-feeding block. By definition everything else is, both literally and figuratively, *inferior* to breast milk and thus no more than a mere basement. And while all infant formulas are breast-milk substitutes, not every breast-milk substitute is an infant formula. Thus, from a nutritional hierarchical (lowerarchical?) standpoint, we can classify formula as the *least-bad* alternative to breast milk and therefore basement 1, even as we might qualify, say, sweetened condensed milk as subbasement 9 and rice-water as subbasement 17 (you're invited to fill in the remaining *subterranean* floors on your own).

If we were to decline to provide our children with the nutritional equivalent of a plush suite in a five-star hotel by feeding them artificially, we would do well not to kid ourselves into believing that, by giving formula, we're somehow at least replacing the suite with adequate three- or four-star accommodation. In fact, our children still end up eating in the basement.

Holding hands with history

Breastfeeding permits us to hold hands simultaneously with yesterday and tomorrow, thereby allowing a little bit of history to pass directly through us today. When a mother who, herself, has been breastfed breastfeeds her child, she at once completes and forges historical links of great consequence. This includes providing a basic blueprint, which is continually responding to the evolving microbial environment, of the very same antibodies that have been in the breast milk of unbroken generations of her female ancestral line even as she passes on this intergenerational potential to any daughters she may bear and nourish.

Row, row your fashion boat

What's your favorite sartorial fantasy? As a male, mine is to be able to walk into Davies & Son, reputed to be the oldest independent tailor (established 1803) on London's storied Savile Row, and order a three-piece bespoke suit and camelhair overcoat out of the finest cloth and interlining. Perhaps yours extends to the high-fashion houses in Paris, for example Chanel, Dior and Lanvin. In either case, unless we win the lottery or Aunt Edith surprises us with a hefty bequest, my guess is that we'll both go on fantasizing while making do with the usual off-the-rack duds. Fortunately, it's not like that with breast milk. We can easily afford to provide our children with the finest in tailor-made nourishment, and this for a fraction of the price of even vulgar mass-produced synthetic nutritional frippery.

Just do your best, Dear

As a child, I was always assured that as long as I did my best in school, all would be well. I didn't have to be first in class. I didn't have to make the honor roll. Theoretically at least, I didn't even have to pass the school year. As long as I did my best, my teachers, and most of all my parents, would be happy. In time, of course, especially after I became a parent myself, I understood the complexity of this disarmingly simple message.

I was of course being prepared for life in the real world and this was meant to cushion the shock of what I would find there. After all, not everyone could attend an elite university (maybe a community college would have to do), step immediately into a high-paying job (Dad wasn't *that* well connected), drive a flashy new luxury car (an ordinary stripped-down used model might be all I could afford), or even be first in line (only one water fountain per floor and more than 40 students per class in my creaky old primary school provided us with an early practical lesson in our thirst for social justice). Fortunately, it's not like that with breast milk. It's true, some parents deliberately opt to provide their children with nutritional mediocrity; but rich or poor, top-of-the-line elite nutrition is accessible to all.

Kinky accoutrements

Imagine for a moment the absurdly successful transformation of the emergency-medical use of an oxygen mask into an everyday must-have fashion accessory. Wouldn't everybody, like, just *so* want to have one? Sure, everyone knows that ambient air is best, but an ambient-air substitute is so cool! And besides, have you seen those adorable unisex plaid- and pastel-motif masks with adjustable headbands and matching canister-carrying back- and fanny-packs – your choice! – that have arrived in the stores just in time for spring?!

In effect, this is what has happened with infant formula. Having started out as a life-saving emergency nutrition intervention, it has migrated from the medicine cabinet to the kitchen pantry. Formula now ranks in the popular mind as just another processed food available at the supermarket. Paradoxically, one of formula's most important comparative advantages in the marketplace is the widespread perception that it's a very close second-best source of nutrition.

The idealized view of infant formula that manufacturers are so adept at portraying – and many ordinary people, health professionals and politicians alike are so disposed to soaking up – translates into a nifty public-relations coup. Moreover, it cleverly avoids any sense of formula's being understood for what it really is – the *least-bad* nutritional alternative to breast milk, whether from a child's own mother, a healthy wet-nurse or a human-milk bank.

In fact, formula manufacturers and their fellow-traveler customers, health professionals and politicians have managed to instill and sustain something which is far more valuable where eating into Mother Nature's market share is concerned – the curious conviction that, while breast is best, infant formula is somehow good enough.

Before you buy shoes, measure your feet (African proverb)

A measurement is only as accurate as the means used to calculate it. The US National Aeronautics and Space Administration contributed a spectacular example of this truism in 1999 when its Mars Climate Orbiter and Mars Polar Lander were destroyed, apparently due to a simple mathematical error. The problem? After investigating, red-faced officials announced preliminary findings. In a critical piece of ground-based navigation software, one development team had used Imperial units, i.e. inches, feet and pounds, while another had used metric units. Since the software hadn't been told to do any conversions, it appeared that the Orbiter got its trajectory wrong and crashed into the Martian surface. Meanwhile, the Mars Polar Lander reached its target at the beginning of December 1999. After 11 months of traveling some 35 million miles (more than 56 million kilometers) in space, the $165 million craft was a mere 130 feet (40 meters) from landing when disaster struck, or rather both the Lander and its piggybacking Deep Space-2 probes were likewise destroyed when they struck the surface.

In one sense, we've been routinely "crash-landing" our babies since the late 1970s by recommending for universal use a growth reference based on a single-community sample of predominantly formula-fed children. The pattern of growth of formula-fed children deviates substantially from that of breastfed children, who grow more rapidly in the first two months and less rapidly, particularly in terms of weight, from three to twelve months. Fortunately, this is changing with the introduction in April 2006 of the new World Health Organization standards for child growth and motor development. They're based on an international sample of nearly 8,500 healthy breastfed children from Brazil, Ghana, India, Norway, Oman and the USA, thereby ensuring ethnic or genetic variability in addition to cultural variation in how children are nurtured. Moreover, the new growth curves provide a single international standard that represents the best description of physiological growth for all children from birth to five years of age while they establish the *breastfed baby* as the normative model for growth and development.

A well-balanced exercise

Breastfeeding is like riding a bicycle built for two. Not only do both front and back riders need to pedal together to permit careful and efficient forward locomotion; they also need to know how to start and stop safely, and of course how to keep their balance in between.

Fortunately, when I was a kid Dad was there to coach and coax me as I learned to ride my very own two-wheeler for the first time. As a result, not only did I have fewer spills, scrapes and scratches than if I'd been on my own, but I also learned the basics of how to guide my own children and grandchildren in this regard many years later. Furthermore, I'm sure that they, too, are now well positioned to pass on this elementary skill information to future generations.

To this day I'm surprised when I meet an adult who admits to having never learned how to ride a bike as a child. How can that be, I wonder. Doesn't *everyone* know?!

Did the Earth move for you, too?

Notwithstanding conventional carnal canons framed in Hollywood storytelling, Harlequin romance novels and bodice-ripper fiction, which of the following options best describes the first time you had sex with a partner?

- Exquisite! The earth moved magically for both of us; we were instantly attuned to meeting each other's every need; and we were totally fulfilled by the experience!
- It was okay but we quickly realized that we still had a lot to learn. So, we promptly resolved to do two things: educate ourselves – and keep doing it until we got it right!
- Frankly disappointing. I remember thinking: Is this all there is?! Too big an investment for too small a gain, really. I might try it again one day, but there's obviously no hurry.
- I found the whole experience disgusting and degrading! I decided, then and there, that flying solo was the way for me. Today, I achieve my pleasure by artificial means only.

Perhaps we need a reference book on the subject of ignorance, including a chapter especially devoted to the generic implications of not knowing what we don't know. What I have in mind is reflected in the all-purpose lament: "I didn't think it was going to be *this* difficult!" – whether "it" refers to riding a bike, having sex or breastfeeding.

Is it the flawed perception that breastfeeding is so utterly intuitive that leads many observers to assume a no-instructions-required attitude in this regard, and then to be surprised that it's "so difficult"? This remarkably common premise – and sure-fire recipe for disappointment and failure – is especially ironic if you consider how lacking in positive breastfeeding role models so much of popular culture is today.

We may in fact be more aware of the challenge of learning to ride a bike or having sex – and more confident in our ability to do both well – than we are of breastfeeding. All three are just as surely natural acts as they are learned behaviors; and even if each is not especially difficult, we still need to know the basics and apply ourselves – until we get it right.

Culture-bound syndromes

When I was an undergraduate majoring in sociology (1965), one of the required courses bore the intriguing title – at least by my barely post-adolescent eyebrow-raising standards – "Sociology of deviant behavior." And I remember well reading one of the course handouts, a cross-cultural comparison of violent crime in just two countries, Japan and the USA. For starters, the criminologist-writer drew up a short list of striking surface similarities between the two, for example income, education, rural/urban population distribution, male/female labor force participation, age structure and life expectancy (all values were virtually indistinguishable from one environment to the other). He then compared the rates between Japan and the USA for three violent crimes: murder, rape and physical assault. You don't need to be a sociologist or for that matter even to have ever set foot in either country – just reasonably well-informed – to figure out what comes next: low to very low rates for these crimes in Japan and high to very high rates in the USA.

As a preface to sharing his views as to why this is so, the criminologist made what initially struck me as an especially outrageous observation: "Having carefully studied the similarities and differences between the two societies, my overall conclusion is that the main problem with violent crime in America is that Americans live there and not Japanese." However, as became quickly clear in reading the remainder of the analysis, what he had in mind was this. Surface similarities notwithstanding, the key cultural qualities that most distinguish Japan from the USA – the dominant other-directed vs. inner-directed cultural norm, and prevailing attitudes toward conflict resolution and delayed vs. immediate satisfaction of individual needs – are the very same qualities that account for citizens' lower or higher propensity to engage in violent behavior. And for the criminologist the implications for reducing the incidence of the three crimes in question in the USA were just as clear. Employing more police, nominating more judges, handing down stiffer prison sentences, building more prisons, and executing still more offenders are not, by themselves, going to have much impact. He then concluded on a fairly pessimistic – but in my view highly perceptive and realistic – note: Until society recognizes and deals in meaningful ways with the *cultural underpinnings* of violence, other action is variously stopgap, reactionary, counterproductive, self-defeating and, in any case, inadequate to carrying the crime-fighting day.

So it is with breastfeeding and our attempts to increase its prevalence and duration. For example, we can wield a variety of blunt instruments like browbeating mothers, using guilt and shame as our prime change-motivating frame of reference, and adding further restrictions to the flow of formula by instituting still more stringent supply-side control measures; or we can roll up our sleeves and attempt to identify – and permanently modify – the cultural underpinnings of the *deviant behavior* that is routine non-emergency artificial feeding.

Historic proportions
American historian Barbara Tuchman published in 1984 what many consider to be her greatest contribution to popular history, *The March of Folly* (New York, Ballantine Books). Here Tuchman analyzes what she considers to be four monumental political blunders committed through the ages in "the blind pursuit of policy contrary to self-interest": the Trojans hauling the wooden horse within their walls some 28 centuries ago, the Renaissance popes provoking the Protestant secession, the 18th-century British attempting to maintain a colonial presence in North America, and what the author labels 20th-century America's self-betrayal in Vietnam.

Tuchman describes four kinds of misgovernment: tyranny of oppression, excessive ambition, incompetence or decadence, and folly or perversity. She concentrates on the last in a specific manifestation – the pursuit of policy contrary to the self-interest of the constituency or state involved. She defines self-interest as "whatever conduces to the welfare or advantage of the body being governed, folly being a policy that in these terms is counterproductive." In addition, she considers her analysis of political folly to be independent of era or locality, timeless and universal, and unrelated to type of regime, nation or class. In a word, she believes her approach to be an archetype of truly universal proportions.

To qualify as folly for her inquiry, the policy adopted must meet three essential criteria: first, it must have been perceived as counterproductive in its own time, not merely in hindsight; second, a feasible alternative course of action must have been available; and to remove the problem from personality a third criterion is that the policy in question should be that of a group, not an individual, and should persist beyond any one political lifetime.

Applying these same criteria to breastfeeding in many environments today, I believe that Tuchman's model provides a startling parallel of indeed historic proportions. Surely, few observers would openly contest that breastfeeding "conduces to the welfare or advantage" of all human society. Likewise, artificial feeding is widely, if hardly unanimously, perceived as counterproductive for the common human good. A feasible alternative course of action to artificial feeding is most assuredly available; it's called breastfeeding. And if we take even a cursory glance at the evolution in society over the last hundred years or so, we recognize that artificial feeding has become the accepted, even expected, child-feeding norm of many groups, thus persisting beyond the lifetime of individuals.

Will breastfeeding, too, one day have its historian-chronicler who tries to unravel the train of events leading to the 20th century's failed mass alternative-nutrition child-feeding trials? And will this same analyst remind her contemporaries of the abundant voices way back in 2006 that clamored for change – as much in public attitudes as in public policy – after meticulous investigation had determined beyond the shadow of a doubt that the unnatural practice of routine non-emergency breast-milk substitution was so irredeemably wanting?

Honor thy mother

Mother Nature doesn't have it all that easy what with so many competitors trying to grab a piece of the child-feeding action. And not only that, as I look around I notice that she's often treated with shocking disrespect: like an old cow by some, like a dumb ass (the kind that's gray, has long ears and eats grass) by others, and like an old goat by still others. But as far as I'm concerned she's more like a thoroughbred bay filly – swift, sleek and sure – and forever a winner. That's why, whenever I step up to the betting window in the Life Long Sweepstakes Office, I always put *my* money on Mother Nature.

The Old man and the bamboo plant

There once was an Old Man who, after a long life of strenuous labor, lived his later years quietly tending, with obvious joy and devotion, the small garden attached to his modest house. The neighbors daily observed him cultivating, fertilizing, primping, pruning, shaping and watering his many bushes, ivies, plants, shoots, shrubs and trees of every type and description.

But of all the garden greenery so lovingly tended, the Old Man paid particular attention to an unusual dwarf-like bamboo plant located in the farthest corner. Daily, he would water it, carefully cultivate and weed the soil around it, and from time to time add a bit of natural fertilizer – all to no visible avail. The neighbors were quick to note that despite his many ministrations it was obvious that the bamboo plant was going nowhere.

Indeed, during the first year there was no change in the plant's physical aspect or disposition; nor was there any alteration well into the second or third years either. This obvious fact gave rise to speculation among some of the Old Man's less-kind neighbors;

perhaps it wasn't a real plant after all but only an ersatz model, albeit a very well-executed one.

Gradually, some neighbors even began to think that the Old Man was having them on, or perhaps that he had "lost it" with age. The least respectful ridiculed him openly, though this had no impact on his continuing devotion to his favorite plant.

On into the fourth year, there was still no visible change, and the neighbors knew, of course, that there never would be. Clearly, the Old Man needed his little joke and most of them considered this a small price to pay to avoid dishonoring a village elder.

Then, suddenly, at the beginning of the fifth year, the bamboo plant began to grow. At first it grew mainly outward, spreading its many luscious leaves in all directions. Very soon, though, it started to shoot upward, too, until it was as tall as the Old Man himself, and then higher still, higher than all the other plants and trees in the entire garden.

Afterward, neighbors saw the Old Man frequently sitting for long periods in the opposite corner, quietly contemplating this marvel of Nature, this mute but verdant testimony to his years of steadfastness.

Now then, are we to assume that the bamboo plant did all its growing during the fifth year only? Or were those earlier years of patient, silent devotion of singular importance as well?

Keeping on keeping on can be a challenge in any human activity – including breastfeeding promotion, especially when we meet with widespread skepticism and fail to observe any apparent change despite our best efforts. We can all use a little encouragement, a gentle reminder that change is often invisible, until one day...

10. Wrapping up and moving on

As a child "mathophobe" regularly reduced to tears in the face of fractions, decimals and long-division, I remember with crystal clarity that stunning breakthrough when, at age 10, I actually grasped, immediately and fully, the significance of the basic algebraic formula: Distance = Speed x Time. I recall that moment today as I contemplate the challenge we face in taking the counterrevolution forward; and this is my conclusion on behalf of the International Breastfeeding Support Collective. Time is really the only fixed variable here since the distance still to be traveled is as irregular as human experience. All that's left for us to adjust then is speed – how quickly our individual acts and collective action, taken together, can increase breastfeeding prevalence and duration. For our children's sake we need to move smartly toward minding more of our own nurturing and nutritional business – and away from other businesses minding them for us. But if you're looking for a comprehensive prescription for change that comes with a guarantee that it will get us where we need to be in record time, I suggest that you're not just reading the wrong book but also probably living on the wrong planet. There can be no universal approach to our universal food and feeding system, which are forever mediated by culture and society. In the process of trying to reconfigure the problem with breastfeeding, I nevertheless feel that some useful conclusions can be drawn to speed things up just a little – and possibly a lot. What do we want Planet Breastfeeding to look like in 2016, 2026, or 2056 when LLLI celebrates its one hundredth anniversary? It's up to the Collective (including you and me) to decide what its goals and objectives should be and then to organize to achieve them. Recalling once again Saul Alinsky's insightful observation, power goes to two poles: to those who've got money and to those who've got people.

I'd like to begin with a recurrent theme of this entire reflection – interconnectedness. We can legitimately assert that Breasts 'R' Us; for human breasts, and the incomparable nurturing and nourishment they provide, help define who and what we are as a species.[1] They also contribute to establishing a species-specific kinship system, both horizontally with the rest of today's human family, and vertically as much with all who have come before us as with all who will come after us. Acting consistently with the biological imperative for feeding the young of our species is thus a universal act of allegiance as much to ourselves as to all our children.

The Collective has its work cut out for it, no doubt about it, if we want to carry these observations to their logical conclusion. To this end, we need to focus more on essentials, on what our real values are or at least what they should be. Those who promote artificial feeding – or who are not all that much troubled when breastfeeding is diminished or ignored – know what values they have in common. Are we entirely clear about ours? In addition to determining which values unite the greatest number, we need to deploy, efficiently and widely, effective arguments using the most suitable language to express and support them.

And even as we continue to think and act locally in the manner most suitable for us as individuals, we need also to think and act globally as members of our universal Collective who are interconnected by a common goal – more and longer breastfeeding – and a common objective – entire societies that are geared to supporting the biological norm for nurturing and nourishing the young of our species. This is globalization with a distinctly happy face.

And speaking of globalization, let's use the Internet more effectively. Let's create the *mother* of all breastfeeding sites, a mega-site of sites, a super-store of the ultimate in accurate and up-to-date scientific, epidemiological, economic and sociocultural information, a portal providing a daily digest of the latest media coverage with an opt-in news-alert facility for e-mail updates, and an easily accessible system for information retrieval. Its purpose: to give Mother Nature the coverage she deserves and to run interference on her behalf when this becomes necessary.

Let's use this site then not only as a source of accurate information but also as a means of tracking down and refuting inaccurate, incomplete, unfounded or otherwise misleading stories, half-truths, false claims or rumors touching on breastfeeding (the abundant sites devoted to nailing down and debunking urban legends provide excellent models for this purpose). Then imagine using the Internet as an effective tool to respond rapidly to the slings, arrows and onslaughts of those who would defy or defile Mother Nature's nurturing and nutritional plan; to track stories, provide topical commentaries, teach and inform, serve as a channel for consumer questions and expert answers; and to link related information sites of all sorts. Separate sections could cover – to mention only a few obvious examples – adopted children, breastfeeding prevalence and duration, breast-milk substitutes, cognitive development, economics, environmental pollutants, epidemiology, ethics, HIV/AIDS, human-milk banking, human rights, legal matters of all sorts, maternal health, morbidity and mortality, oral health, and the workplace, each with its own dynamic Q&A component built up over time in response to real-world experience.

Let's call this mega-site Planet Breastfeeding. In fact, although I have no intention of developing it myself, I've already registered www.planetbreastfeeding.org as a domain name; what's more, I'm prepared to turn it over to the right person or persons – defined as those presenting a responsible, credible and sustainable plan for making it happen. The goal would be for the site to be available in all six official languages of the United Nations – initially in at least English, French and Spanish and later in Arabic, Chinese and Russian – and in as many other languages as resources and size of viewing public permit. If the right organizing tactics and promotional skills are used, funding this unique global information resource should not present insurmountable difficulties. Sponsors could be a broad-based consortium drawn from the Collective's current membership including private individuals, groups and foundations, and international nongovernmental, health professional and intergovernmental organizations.

Let's make sure that this mega-site champions only Mother Nature, in other words that it focuses on no one else's or any other group's interests or agenda no matter how noble or worthy of support. To achieve this, the consortium would need to nominate an independent multidisciplinary board of directors, an international council of wise persons, with each member serving a maximum set number of years.

Let's imagine the site serving like a combined referral hospital with its full complement of services, and a specialty hospital dedicated to providing focused specific care. "Patients" would be regularly referred to the Mother site for major "interventions" or when sophisticated "intensive care" facilities were required, and also back again to the myriad other linked sites run by groups and individuals – currently numbering a potential 8.5 million according to Google when searching with the single key word "breastfeeding".

We have more than adequate information to reaffirm energetically the numerous benefits of breast milk and breastfeeding, even if "everyone" supposedly already knows this. But it's time we also emphasized the steadily expanding evidence about the short- and longer-term risks associated with routine artificial feeding; they should surprise no one given so fundamental a deviation from the biological norm for the young of our species. I propose this be done initially by undertaking major multi-center research projects, in representative low-, medium- and high-income settings, followed by international expert consultations to present results and forge global consensus on two interrelated topics:

Topic one: "Beyond breast is best" – to focus on the multiple risks of artificial feeding and their impact on the health of children and mothers alike, and thus society as a whole, throughout the life course.

Topic two: "We can't afford not to breastfeed" – to get a firm fix on the multiple, complex and lifelong economic implications of observing or disregarding the hominid blueprint for nourishing the young of our species.

And for the sake of infants who have to be fed on a breast-milk substitute, let's also review the available evidence – or generate new information as required – concerning the nutritional adequacy of infant formula and the period during which formula alone can be said to meet babies' nutritional needs, which is also to say when complementary feeding should begin for babies who are deprived of breast milk. WHO undertook such a systematic review for breast milk in 2000-2001,[2] but it has never conducted a comparable inquiry for infant formula even if the norm of four-to-six-months nutritional adequacy has been in place since the late 1970s.[3]

Between the systematic review and the recommendations of an international expert consultation,[4] and now the results of the Multicentre Growth Reference Study and the new WHO Growth Reference Standards,[5] for the first time in nutritional history we've at last got the goods on Mother Nature. It's about time we had a better fix on the competition, prepared in the same disinterested way, which is to say by those who don't stand to benefit financially from the outcome. But we need to be prepared to deal with the inevitable political objections to this exercise, as if looking at the nutritional adequacy of formula – and thus how possibly to make formula less inadequate – somehow implied endorsing its routine use. Think again of helping to ensure safety on board ships and airplanes with appropriate equipment, for use *in case of emergency*. This hardly suggests a disaster or death wish, quite the contrary.

Meanwhile, as debate continues[6] on revision of the Codex Standard for Infant Formula (originally adopted in 1976),[7] some knowledgeable observers have concluded that commercial interests may in fact be the strongest driver of exactly what and how much goes inside.[8] Particular attention has been drawn to the absence of scientific arguments for the approach the International Dairy Federation is advocating (with support from several Codex member states with strong dairy industries) for determining infant formula protein; and a controversial method for setting maximum values for nutrients that flouts the "guiding principle [that] infant formulas should contain components only in such amounts that serve a nutritional purpose, provide another benefit, or are necessary for technological reasons." In the view of these observers, contrary to strong scientific advice, "some member states requested that maximum values should be established only for levels of nutrients with documented adverse effects in infants, while in all other cases only interim values should be established which would not be binding for manufacturers." These critics conclude their arguments by advising that "doctors should choose and recommend only those infant formulas with compositions based on current scientific knowledge and on the nutritional requirements of infants."[9]

Let's establish networks, and then let's establish networks of networks, inventively using a cascading-coalition principle. For example, we can invite obstetricians/gynecologists, pediatricians, family physicians, midwives, neonatal nurses, nutritionists, dietitians, lactation consultants, health visitors and other support workers to participate – first as individuals, then through their national, regional and international associations, and finally as members of broad-based health-professional alliances. All these groups, too, could contribute to swelling the ranks of the Collective's grand coalition.

Let's also combine our forces with appropriate national and international associations in related areas, for example breast-cancer prevention and the promotion of oral health. This includes national cancer and dental societies of course, but also the International Agency for Research on Cancer[10] and the International Association for Dental Research[11] among other international bodies. All parties should be providing the same basic information, the same consistent convergent message – breastfeeding protects the health of mothers and children alike. However, for the most part both national and international organizations in these two vital areas of human health promotion and disease prevention remain strangely silent on these vital issues, while privately funded groups have a decidedly mixed record in this regard (see entries on breastfeeding and cancer risk reduction in chapter 5). Fortunately, at least in respect to oral health promotion, reliable sources like LLLI[12] and dedicated private practitioners like Brian Palmer[13] fill the information gap to a degree. But this glaring lack of common purpose, information sharing and synergy, nationally and internationally, is a prime example of a major missed collaborative opportunity that cries out for the Collective's urgent attention.

Let's draw in other partners with small but nevertheless potentially important roles to play, for example the International Organization for Standardization (ISO),[14] which is the world's leading developer of standards designed to be implemented worldwide; and the Airports Council International (ACI),[15] which is the "voice of the world's airports". Both organizations could contribute to global acceptance of breastfeeding as the child-feeding norm, the former by developing and promoting, as the global standard, suitable signs, symbols and ideograms – for example mother-and-baby line drawings in lieu of the ubiquitous back-lit feeding bottle – and the latter for advocating prominent placement of these emblems, as a uniform testimony to normality, to indicate to the world's traveling public where child-care facilities can be found in the more than 1,600 airports in 177 countries and territories of ACI's 569 members.

To community-based mother-support groups everywhere I have this to say: You are not just invited to participate in this grand coalition; you are asked to help lead it! After all, it is you who have labored so long, so hard, and so often in forced isolation, particularly during the last half-century, to keep the breastfeeding flame burning brightly while much of the rest of society looked the other way. And it is you who have played so significant a role in many settings not only in terms of arresting breastfeeding's decline but also in turning prevalence and duration rates around. Please continue to do for all our mothers and children what other mothers of good will and huge heart have done for each other since pre-history. And may your ordinary daily miracles continue to inspire the rest of us to contribute in every possible way.

And if I were in a position to speak to the world's governments, this is what I would say: As guarantors of the welfare of your citizens, you of course will want to move beyond reciting pious breast-is-best slogans and adopting, through your international organizations, still more resolutions, declarations, strategies and plans of action that essentially reiterate what has already been said over and over for the last 30 years. You of course will want to concentrate your energy and resources on implementing, systematically and fully, those remarkably sound and comprehensive consensus instruments that are *already* on the table.[16] And as you know, the scientific and epidemiological evidence on which these instruments are so firmly based is both unassailable and expanding daily.

The welfare of your citizens is at this price, and the health of your economies depends on it much more than you probably know. Just ask your health economists to take a wide-ranging and comprehensive look at the question. Focusing narrowly for a moment to make the point: We're not just talking about less diarrhea[17] and respiratory tract infection[18] here; we're also looking at significantly higher scores for cognitive development.[19] Brains are forever![20] Be honest now. What do you suppose is the cumulative worth, over a lifetime, of 5 to 10 points[21] on an IQ scale for every child-citizen born within your national territory?[22]

For governments of resource-poor countries in particular, I would like to recall why you began taking action in the 1980s to combat iodine deficiency, which is the world's single most common cause of mental retardation and brain damage. It happened when you understood the size of this massive public health problem – with 2.2 billion people, or 38% of the world's population, living in areas of iodine deficiency – and its implications for brain development, and therefore the educability and economic productivity of your citizens.[23] Given the impact of faulty feeding practices on postpartum brain development, how could you possibly hesitate to take all-out action now in support of breastfeeding?

And let's not forget breastfeeding's role in lowering significantly the risk of morbidity and mortality among your children; and in protecting the health of your mothers, including by reducing the risk of postpartum hemorrhaging and anemia, increasing the time between pregnancies (thanks to lactational amenorrhea), reducing the overall number of pregnancies (due to a greater number of surviving children) and thereby enhancing the health and well-being of mothers and children alike.

By the way – and I'm addressing all governments here – have you given any thought to juxtaposing your national breastfeeding rate at six months, your infant mortality rate[24] and your incarceration rate[25] to see what correlations you might observe? Ironically, you may well find that, of the three datasets, breastfeeding rates at six months are the least easy to come by.

And if I had the chance, these are some of the things that I would say to intergovernmental organizations: You need to be more aware of the implicit generic contract between speakers and listeners, writers and readers, on any topic. While one is responsible primarily for what is said or written the other is responsible primarily for what is heard or read. But if, at the outset, the message is incomplete, unclear, confused, incoherent or distorted – where does the burden lie then?

For example, what exactly do you mean when you say that, globally, an estimated 3,500 lives could be saved *each day* if every baby were exclusively breastfed for the first six months of life?[26] Have you made very sure that the relative-rich reading this copy understand what is being discussed here – the lives of precisely which babies, where and why? Because if they don't you risk confusing readers, not being taken seriously or, worse, being dismissed as liars. (I reacted similarly to the obviously positive news out of Ghana[27] (see chapter 6) about how breastfeeding in the first *hour* of life could save the lives of almost one million babies each year). Please understand: I'm not calling these numbers into question; on the contrary, I suspect they might even be on the low side, but that's not my point.

Raw numbers, served cold and unqualified like this, can result in more than incredulity; for the uninformed, they can contribute to the perverse conclusion that, unlike people living in poverty, the relative rich are somehow able to feed their children fret-free formula. After all, in resource-rich settings artificially fed babies aren't exactly dying in the streets; their added morbidity and mortality are found – or, given confounders like access to medical services, in fact hidden – elsewhere. What we already know about breastfeeding's dose-response[28] in terms of lowering morbidity and mortality in *all* settings should be adequate to motivate governments everywhere to take a closer look at artificial feeding's negative short- and longer-term impact on their populations; but this will not happen, either in rich countries or among elites in poor countries, if the wrong messages are taken up.

And recalling my earlier implied request to governments: Intergovernmental organizations are of course urged to take any new action that may be called for to protect, promote and support breastfeeding. But please hold off on adopting still more resolutions, declarations, strategies and plans of action that only duplicate what has already been said repeatedly. Concentrate instead on systematically implementing the consensus instruments *already* on the table.

And the infant-food industry – does it have a place at the table? Yes, I think it does, albeit a narrowly defined ad hoc one, in the same way that manufacturers of *emergency* equipment – for example air bags, oxygen masks, life vests and inflatable rafts – have places at consortium tables around which also sit hospitals, airlines, aircraft and automobile manufacturers, accident prevention bureaus and consumer organizations. I'm not naively suggesting that the infant-food industry, as presently self-perceived, will *voluntarily* assume such a narrowly defined and spartan straight-back chair in favor of its currently coveted cushy one; just that, if this is indeed the seat we want the industry to occupy, it's up to us to effect the downward product-demand shift – through significantly more and longer breastfeeding – that will make industry only too glad to grab it out of sheer enlightened self-interest. But as with gradually shifting society-wide attitudes toward tobacco and in recent decades, we're not going to see this downward shift in product demand happen overnight, or at all, except by altering the way society *as a whole* views artificial feeding and its life-long negative consequences.

And since I'm speaking about the infant-food industry, this is what I would say to its representatives if I were given the opportunity: It seems to me that your choices are clear if not particularly palatable:

- You could continue operating under your own special brand of denial, dragging your corporate feet for, at most, the next 15 to 20 years while doing your best to slow the slide in sales of your myriad infant-formula products, which are intended for routine non-emergency use, by seeking to subvert the switch to more and longer breastfeeding (indeed, given the principles traditionally governing profit-making, this is what you'd be expected to do); *or* you could defy tradition by preparing for changed consumer behavior resulting from increasing society-wide awareness of breastfeeding's essential nurturing and nutritional role.

- You could demonstrate yet again that you're really not interested in what breastfeeding proponents have to say, only in working as close as possible to the margins of enforced regulations; that you have no intention of accepting the prospect of less profit without a fight; and that, instead, you will continue pushing for as much profit as possible today and adapt only at the last moment to changes in market conditions tomorrow; *or* you could reconsider your position in the cold light of that fabled sine qua non of commercial acumen – a hard-nosed assessment of the enlightened self-interest just referred to above.

- You could willfully stay *behind* the curve, continuing merrily doing whatever you manage to get away with in terms of what today's market will bear, only having to scramble, in tomorrow's, to cope with the inevitable shift in consumer demand resulting from an incrementally successful counterrevolution (due primarily to the increased prevalence and duration of breastfeeding, but also including multiplication of non-profit human-milk banks in high-, middle- and low-income countries (see chapter 4) to meet mushrooming special-needs demand, for example to feed preterm and low-birth-weight babies and those abandoned or orphaned due to HIV/AIDS); *or* you could opt to move *ahead* of the curve by preparing for tomorrow when at least a few of your products will still be needed, albeit in significantly reduced quantity and frequency.

So, welcome to the table; but before you take your seat I'd like to make sure you understand that you're invited here based on the Collective's exceedingly narrow definition of your role. You see, the common ground we promote is *naturally* weighted in favor of breastfeeding; and because we believe there really is no place for routine, non-emergency artificial feeding *anywhere*, you should also know that the Collective considers *intrinsically unethical* any attempt to compete with Mother Nature by seeking to diminish her market share in favor of a synthetic substitute typically, though not exclusively, based on the milk of an alien species.

Breastfeeding and breast milk are ideas whose time has returned. As an industry, you habitually pride yourselves as being at the vanguard in terms of anticipating and responding rapidly to consumer needs. Here's your chance to prove it by jumping in *today* on the right side of history. How cool is that?

But I'm not exactly holding my breath. As I said earlier, given the principles traditionally governing profit-making, putting the interests of mothers and children first is not at all what you'd be expected to do spontaneously. Please note: Whatever you decide, you will henceforth no longer be able to say that you were never warned about the consequences if you don't.

This century belongs to breastfeeding!

Where health professionals responsible for caring for mothers and children are concerned, this is what I would say if I were given the opportunity: I have enormous respect for your knowledge, training and hard-won experience, but I have zero understanding or tolerance for any fence-sitting you may still be engaging in concerning breast milk and breastfeeding. If you have a cultural blind spot or two to overcome, that's fine; go ahead and do it. After all, your health degree doesn't make you any less a product of the larger society and culture in which you were born, came of age and were educated. But do you really think you have a valid excuse for not coming down routinely on Mother Nature's side? If so, I wonder what it might be. It seems to me that the abundant, readily available, and overwhelmingly clear and convincing scientific and epidemiological evidence speaks for itself – and certainly a lot louder than I can.

As a group you are seen as authorities on every aspect of maternal and child care and nutrition; thus you are in a unique position to influence the organization and functioning of health services for mothers before, during and after pregnancy and delivery, which of course is what the successfully implemented Baby-friendly Hospital Initiative is all about.[29] But health professionals who are knowledgeable about breastfeeding and motivated to promote it energetically don't fall from the sky. Further upstream you and your professional associations and training institutions need to ensure that appropriate teaching curricula and policies are in place so that all members of all related professions are actively prepared to protect, promote and support breastfeeding as they should.

Yet, as a group or individually, you may still not be doing enough of the right things or you may even be actively doing too many of the wrong things. I'm struck by the disquieting tendency in some settings for health professionals to abstain from providing much advice, let alone a considered opinion, on feeding, as if a "whatever you think is best" approach were a satisfactory way to meet the needs of the mothers and babies you are privileged to serve. Is this linked to a misplaced desire not to offend or inflict guilt? (If so, don't bother telling parents they shouldn't smoke or that they should protect their children against the main childhood diseases, use an approved car-seat to transport them, and keep medicines and cleaning products out of their reach.) Or is it more an extension of the so-called politically correct or highly litigious society in which some of you find yourselves, where finally no one dares take a stand anymore on much of anything? I don't know what the answer is or, more likely, what the answers are. But my sense is that it's time for some plain thinking and plain talking here among health professionals – and for any stragglers to climb quickly down off the child-feeding fence directly on the side of history.

Lastly, as you strive to serve mothers and babies, perhaps you would like to reflect on the following: the possible relevance, for your attitude toward the original default food and feeding system, of what philosopher and social critic Ivan Illich had to say about experts and professionalization:

> *The medical establishment has become a major threat to health. The case against expert systems like modern health care is that they can produce a damage which outweighs potential benefits; they obscure the political conditions that render society unhealthy; and they tend to expropriate the power of individuals to heal themselves and to shape their environments.*[30]

And while I have your attention, I'd like to invite you to join me in declaring a moratorium on using the overworked, unhelpful and often misappropriated slogan "breast is best"; or perhaps we could even agree to banish it altogether from our collective vocabulary.

My final observations are directed toward breastfeeding advocates in general, including me of course. If we're not careful, we can easily come across to some mothers as if insisting that we're the only ones knowledgeable about feeding children and that they should just keep quiet and dutifully follow our instructions. My superficially paradoxical response here is that we need to be both more aggressive – that is more rigorous – within the Collective and less aggressive – by acting always with generosity and humility – in our dealings with those who have not yet joined. We also need to be aware of the pitfalls of the expert trap:

> *Experts and an expert culture always call for more experts. Experts also have a tendency to cartelize themselves by creating 'institutional barricades' – for example proclaiming themselves gatekeepers, as well as self-selecting themselves. Finally, experts control*

> knowledge production, as they decide what valid and
> legitimate knowledge is, and how its acquisition is
> sanctioned.[31]

I also suggest that we reflect on the intrinsic properties of sugar and vinegar – and the adage about attracting more flies with the former than with the latter. There will always be examples of "cultural lag," which is the term behavioral scientists use to describe a slower rate of change in one part of society compared with another. So, said simply, some mothers still need more time to catch up. Browbeating them is at best counterproductive for today and, at worst, counterproductive for always. Meanwhile, of course, we should be unrelenting in our efforts to re-shape culture, and society and its institutions, to ensure not only that mothers, because they are *genuinely* informed, choose breastfeeding every time, but also that they are fully supported in their choice.

Taking a long look at history, I sometimes have the impression that few topics have been as thoroughly obscured by unsound information, contradictory beliefs and illogical thinking as child feeding. Yet I don't think it would be excessively boastful if I were to affirm that we are collectively becoming ever more knowledgeable ... about our ignorance. The key messages are clearer now: that during the early years the nurturing role of mothers is central to children's healthy physical, intellectual and emotional development; and that babies are indeed born to be breastfed. Neither nurturing nor nourishing naturally can be entirely safely substituted; the best we can hope to accomplish is to minimize the inherent risks.

I'll put it this way. In light of 200 million or so years of mammalian evolution,[32] we're finally beginning to see routine recourse to the paltry pay-off of a century and a half of laboratory fiddling for what it really is: monumental short-sighted scientific hubris. Whether growing awareness of our ignorance and the hard-won scientific facts accompanying it will be enough to influence political and economic events, and thereby markedly improve global society's child-feeding practices, remains to be seen. Attempts to derive social policy from biological concepts are not risk-free. Yet, as we have learned – both in terms of the benefits of breastfeeding and the risks of artificial feeding – the alternative conjures up a truly appalling vision of nurturing and nutritional mediocrity for children, mothers and society as a whole.

I consider myself an optimist by nature and this surely extends to breastfeeding, whether protecting it where it's still the norm or promoting it where it's not. And I remain convinced that, as the traditional civil rights anthem affirms, we shall indeed overcome – one day. It's mainly a question of how quickly the Collective can move the counterrevolution forward. I'm not so foolhardy to assume that I have the answer; but I've tried in these pages to stimulate your thinking about how we might at least formulate the most relevant questions while reconfiguring, and candidly considering, the *real* problem with breastfeeding.

As members of the International Breastfeeding Support Collective, we have considerable potential for effecting positive change even if, by itself, this is no guarantee of our ultimate success. As cartoonist-philosopher Charles Schulz tidily sums up the human condition through the plaintive words of his little *Peanuts* pal Linus: "There's no heavier burden than a great potential."[33] It really is time for us to move on, all together, in pursuit of ours.

References

1. All mammals share at least three characteristics not found in other animals: middle ear bones, hair and the production of milk by modified sweat glands called mammary glands. Myers P, Wund M. Animal Diversity Web, University of Michigan Museum of Zoology, Class Mammalia http://animaldiversity.ummz.umich.edu/site/accounts/information/Mammalia.html.

2. The optimal duration of exclusive breastfeeding. A systematic review. Geneva, World Health Organization, 2001 http://www.who.int/nutrition/publications/optimal_duration_of_exc_bfeeding_review_eng.pdf.

3. Background technical document for the Joint WHO/UNICEF Meeting on Infant and Young Child Feeding (October 9-12, 1979). World Health Organization, Geneva, 1979.

4. The optimal duration of exclusive breastfeeding. Report of an Expert Consultation. Geneva, World Health Organization, 2001 http://www.who.int/nutrition/publications/optimal_duration_of_exc_bfeeding_report_eng.pdf.

5. The WHO Multicentre Growth Reference Study (MGRS) http://www.who.int/childgrowth/mgrs/en/.

6. Codex Committee on Nutrition and Foods for Special Dietary Uses, 28th Session, Chiang Mai, Thailand, October 30 - November 3, 2006.

7. Codex Alimentarius. *Codex standard 72 on infant formula* (CODEX STAN 72-1981) http://www.codexalimentarius.net/download/standards/288/CXS_072e.pdf. Amended in 1985, 1987 and 1997.

8. Koletzko B, Raanan S. Standards for infant formula milk. Commercial interests may be the strongest driver of what goes into formula milk. *British Medical Journal*, 2006, 332:621-622.

9. Ibid.

10. The International Agency for Research on Cancer http://www.iarc.fr/ is part of the World Health Organization. Located in Lyon, France, IARC's mission is to coordinate and conduct research on the causes of human cancer and the mechanisms of carcinogenesis, and to develop scientific strategies for cancer control.

11. The mission of the International Association for Dental Research is to advance research and increase knowledge for the improvement of oral health worldwide http://www.dentalresearch.org/about/iadr/mission.html.

12. La Leche League International, Schaumburg, Illinois. Breastfeeding and Dental Health http://www.lalecheleague.org/NB/NBdental.html.

13. Brian Palmer, D.D.S. For better Health! http://www.brianpalmerdds.com/.

14. International Organization for Standardization http://www.iso.org/iso/en/aboutiso/isoinbrief/isoinbrief.html, P.O. Box 56, 1211 Geneva 20, Switzerland.

15. Airports Council International, P.O. Box 16, 1215 Geneva 15 - Airport, Switzerland http://www.airports.org/cda/aci/display/main/aci_content.jsp?zn=aci&cp=1-2^4382_9_2__.

16. The most obvious is the most recent and the most comprehensive, the Global Strategy for Infant and Young Child Feeding, op. cit.

17. Howie PW et al. Protective effect of breast feeding against infection. Op. cit.; Quigley MA, Cumberland P, Cowden JM, Rodrigues LC. How protective is breast feeding against diarrhoeal disease in infants in 1990s England? A case-control study. *Archives of Disease in Childhood*, 2006, 91:245-250.

18. Chantry CJ, Howard CR, Auinger P. Full breastfeeding duration and associated decrease in respiratory tract infection in US children. *Pediatrics*, 2006, 117(2):425-432.

19. Anderson JW, Johnstone BM, Remley DT. Breast-feeding and cognitive development: a meta-analysis. *American Journal of Clinical Nutrition*, 1999, 70(4):525-535.

20. As Nils Bergman (Senior Medical Superintendent, Mowbray Maternity Hospital, Cape Town. South Africa) describes it: "Breastfeeding is a behavior which shapes and sculpts the brain, and that brain shaping stays for life. Skin-to-skin contact is what the newborn requires in order for the brain to be shaped in the best possible way, and breastfeeding in the fullest sense is not about eating, but about brain growth, and the development of good relationships. Any other form of care is experienced by the newborn as separation, and prolonged separation causes permanent harm to babies' brains." Health Promotion Agency for Northern Ireland, Press Release, May 17, 2005, *All-island breastfeeding conference highlights significant health impact of breastfeeding*.

21. Daniels MC, Adari LS. Breast-feeding influences cognitive development in Filipino children. *Journal of Nutrition*, 2005, 135:2589-2595.

22. Lawlor DA et al. Early life predictors of childhood intelligence: findings from the Mater-University study of pregnancy and its outcomes. Op. cit.

23. International Council for the Control of Iodine Deficiency Disorders, IDD Problem Statement http://indorgs.virginia.edu/iccidd/aboutidd.htm#problem.

24. The World Factbook, Rank Order – Infant mortality rate (data as of 10 January 2006) http://www.cia.gov/cia/publications/factbook/rankorder/2091rank.html.

25. King's College London, International Centre for Prison Studies. World Prison Population List (sixth edition), June 2005, http://www.kcl.ac.uk/depsta/rel/icps/world-prison-population-list-2005.pdf.

26. UNICEF. Breastfeeding can save over 1 million lives yearly. Press Release, New York, July 30, 2004 http://www.unicef.org/media/media_22646.html.

27. Edmond KM et al. Delayed breastfeeding initiation increases risk of neonatal mortality. Op. cit.

28. Dose response, which applies to individuals or to populations, is the change in effect on an organism caused by differing levels of exposure to a substance. This is aptly illustrated by the recent secondary analysis of data from a nationally representative cross-sectional home survey conducted from 1988 to 1994 in the USA showing that infants who were fully breastfed for 4 months to <6 months were at more than four times greater risk of pneumonia and twice the risk of otitis media than those who were fully breastfed for ≥6 months. See: Chantry CJ, Howard CR, Auinger P. op. cit.

29. Merewood A, Mehta SD, Chamberlain LB, Philipp BL, Bauchner H. Breastfeeding rates in US baby-friendly hospitals: results of a national survey. *Pediatrics*, 2005, 116(3):628-634; UNICEF UK Baby Friendly Initiative. Baby Friendly Initiative increases breastfeeding rates in Switzerland, December 13, 2005 http://www.babyfriendly.org.uk/mailing/updates/research_update_20051213.htm; Swissinfo. Breastfeeding wins mothers' approval, January 12, 2006 http://swissinfo.org/sen/swissinfo.html?siteSect=107&sid=6377171&cKey=1137059875000.

30. Illich I. *Medical Nemesis: The expropriation of health*, London, Marian Boyars, 1975.

31. Finger M, Asún JM. *Adult Education at the Crossroads. Learning our way out*. London, Zed Books, 2001.

32. Estimates of the number of mammals (4500-5500) and when the first mammals appeared vary depending on the source of information and approach to classification used. The Web site *Welcome to the incredible world of mammals* http://www.earthlife.net/mammals/welcome.html states that "the first mammals appeared about 265 million years ago, a mere 10 million years after the first dinosaurs, but they remained relatively obscure for the first 160 million years while the dinosaurs ruled". The site goes on to say: "The first mammal may never be known, but the Genus *Morganucodon* and in particular *Morganucodon watsoni*, a 2-3 cm (1 inch) long weasel-like animal whose fossils were first found in caves in Wales and around Bristol (UK), but later unearthed in China, India, North America, South Africa and Western Europe is a possible contender. It is believed to be between 200 MYA [million years ago] and 210 MYA. However *Gondwanadon tapani* reported from India on the basis of a single tooth in 1994 may be an earlier contender for the title, with a claimed date of 225 MYA."

33. Schulz CM. Linus on life. New York: Hallmark Cards Inc., 1965.

Index

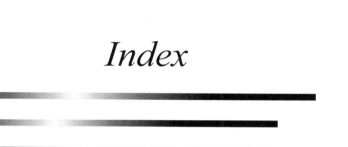

James Akre was born in the USA where he lived until the age of 21, including four years on a Pennsylvania dairy farm which was part of the secondary school complex he attended. His international career began as an adviser to rural populations in Turkey (1966) and Cameroon (1968) in small animal husbandry and farmer cooperatives. After obtaining his master's degree in economic and social development 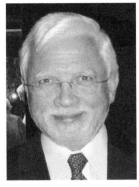 (University of Pittsburgh, 1972), he worked for more than 30 years with various international organizations focusing on labor and social affairs; technical and material support to the agriculture, education and public health sectors in low-income countries; and public health nutrition, with particular emphasis on feeding infants and young children. He currently serves as a member of the International Board of Lactation Consultant Examiners. Jim and his Swiss wife Pia, who is a primary-school health educator, live in Geneva, Switzerland; they have two daughters and a son, and three grandchildren. Besides writing, Jim enjoys running, sailing, photography, and singing classical and contemporary choral works as a member of the Geneva Amateur Operatic Society.

Ordering Information

Hale Publishing, L.P.
1712 N. Forest St.
Amarillo, Texas 79106, USA

8:00 am to 5:00 pm CST

Call...806-376-9900
Sales...800-378-1317
FAX...806-376-9901

International (+1-806)-376-9900

Online Web Orders...
http://www.iBreastfeeding.com